man's common sense

GUIDE TO PHYSICAL FITNESS

man's common sense

GUIDE TO PHYSICAL FITNESS

ROBERT DELMONTEQUE

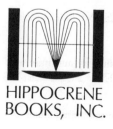

HIPPOCRENE
BOOKS, INC.

HIPPOCRENE BOOKS, INC.
171 Madison Avenue • New York 10016

Distributed by Optimum Book Marketing, Inc.

Library of Congress catalog number 72-84062

ISBN 0 88254 021 1

Published by arrangement with
FRED KERNER / PUBLISHING PROJECTS

Printed in the United States of America

Author's Introduction

You no longer have to diet on rabbit food, or follow an Olympic weightlifting schedule, to keep your waistline down and your strength up. You need no other equipment, or props, than what you have in your house or apartment—or hotel room, for that matter.

In the brief instructions and simple guidelines that follow, I have set out for you a program so elementary and concise that its demands —in point of time and discomfort—will be about equal to the period you spend brushing your teeth and shaving each morning.

The content of this book has one magnificent asset: It works!

The principles you will learn here have been proved again and again. Using them I have lost a million pounds, to the great relief and good health of thousands of men. Many of the exercises in this book may seem familiar to you. Some of the comments on food may have a second-time ring. There are no new discoveries in body manipulation, for the very good reason that they are not needed. There are no magic oils you can drink to melt the fat away and there won't be, until one of Ponce de Leon's men emerges from the Everglades with a good map leading back to the fountain.

No, the principles in this book are not new; except in the sense that nobody seems to know about them. They have never before been put into a sensible, practical plan for the average Joe.

Volumes have been written in the past few years, picturing every conceivable type of exercise. Even more has been written in the name of *Diet,* which has become a harsh four-letter word in our vocabulary. All of these essays have two faults in common:

1) They tell you more than you want to know.

2) They demand too much of you.

So this book was written to fill the need for a no-nonsense streamlined guide to physical fitness and normal weight. There is no wasted motion nor wasted time in this direct line to good health and a longer life.

This shortcut has one basic secret, which I have discovered in a quarter century of study and practical application:

Every man, either overweight or underweight, needs *his own individual* conditioning program.

Once he has it, the rest is simple.

I have been forced to find a workable way for men to lose weight and build muscle. If I hadn't, I suppose I would be out selling insurance like 90 per cent of the other men in this country. I have been a lecturer, writer, calisthenics-shouter—in short, pretty much on an all-around health kick all the 44 years of my life. I escaped from Muscle Beach long ago to begin taking a practical approach to physical fitness for the businessman, the junior executive, the ex-athletes and the non-athletes. It was in Europe, for the moneyed members of health clubs in Paris and Rome, that I first set up the Delmonteque System for exercise and weight loss. I do the same thing now, in a more substantial way, at luxury clubs throughout the Southwest.

The members of these clubs come in all shapes and sizes, all ages, and in various states of physical fitness—or unfitness. Included is astronaut Alan Shepard, who has been shot out of the Cape Kennedy cannon, perfect physical specimen. A dozen of the astronauts are members of the Houston club, including the new group whose names are marked for future headlines—Charley Conrad, Frank Borman, Jim McDivitt, Jim Lovell and Tom Stafford.

What possible set of exercises could benefit, or even be possible, for all the club members, astronauts as well as ageing business executives? There is none, of course. Yet they all fitted neatly into the

Delmonteque system and they all achieved the results they sought. There are thousands more, readers of my newspaper columns in Houston, Dallas, Indianapolis and 36 other cities across the country, who have had similar success. Every day a letter arrives from someone recounting a new story. These are men, even as you, who want to regain the shape of their lost youth. All they needed was a workable plan.

This book will spell out your own individual program, and then it will go beyond that to the dozens of personal foibles which may or may not plague you. Has it been your fondest dream since boyhood to "make a muscle" and display a 16-inch bicep? It's not too late. A scrawny neck, or a roll of fat spilling over your collar? Easily solved. You'll discover the exercise that Hollywood's western he-men use to keep those bags from under their eyes. We will examine the case against cholesterol as a contributor to heart disease, how to stave off baldness and even grayness, how to get a good night's sleep, and how to relieve desk-bound tensions at the office.

Only rarely do I find there's something I have overlooked, or some way I have failed to get the complete message across, as I failed recently in the case of one of the most fabled members of the Houston club, Glenn McCarthy. McCarthy was the boy-wonder king of the wildcatters who opened up the last big oil bonanza in Texas. His two-fisted Irish personality has always been as rich as his personal fortune, and The McCarthy has never been too far out of shape, even now as the entrepreneur of the $1 million penthouse Cork Club and the promoter of his own bourbon, Wildcatter.

McCarthy tore into the Delmonteque system with a wild cry, but for six mysterious weeks he got nowhere. In fact, he gained a few pounds. In the seventh week, I felt the nudge of his temper.

"Bob," he said, in his soft and steely voice, "looks like you've been handing me a lot of baloney with all this exercise and food stuff. Nothing's happening."

"If you've been following your program," I said, "you have to be making progress."

"I've been following the blankety-blank program. Right down the line. And nothing."

I said, "Calm yourself, Glenn. Let's sit down and talk this thing over. You must be picking up some hidden calories somewhere."

We went over McCarthy's meals for the past week, and he'd done even better than I expected. I knew that he was on a good exercise program because we had a record of his performance. Finally, I said, "What about liquids?"

"Well—," McCarthy thought a moment. "I have a bottle of wine with lunch and a bottle of wine with dinner, and a bottle of Wildcatter bourbon in between. Any calories in that?"

man's common sense

GUIDE TO PHYSICAL FITNESS

The Happy Shortcut to Losing Weight

Let's face it. What you want is to get in shape through very little effort. You want to lose weight and regain some of your old vigor. But you are repelled by the notion of personal sacrifice and such hostile words as Hard Work, and Will Power.

You know that the art of reducing can be broken down into two methods: 1) It is possible to lose weight, while pursuing your regular eating habits, by strenuous programs of formal exercise, or 2) it is possible to lose weight, while exerting no more energy than you do now, by cutting food intake down to starvation levels.

Well, relax. Just so we'll understand each other, let's take it for granted that you score very low on Will Power where your physical self is concerned and that you already have your share of Hard Work at your job.

Happily, there is a third method in the art of reducing which logically borrows from the first two. If you exercise a little *and* change your eating habits a little, you can shed pounds like a snowman in the sun. The two factors multiply each other, the exercise burning away that spare tire around your middle, and solid menus restoring your energy for more exercise.

Even the word *Exercise* is not the tough baby you think it is. Let's clear away the major misconceptions on the subject right now:

It is punishing. False. Somehow the notion got around that exercise has to hurt a little before it can do you "any good." This is not only foolishness, but downright dangerous. Each of the exercises in this book have the constant proviso that you work inside your own capacity.

Discomfort is required. False. The Spartan notions that you must perform exercises on a rock-hard floor, in a drafty or stifling gymnasium, or that the crack of dawn is the only worthwhile time of day —all of these ideas cause a lot of needless pain and wasted effort. Each exercise is focused on one particular area of the body. The rest of you can take it easy.

It increases your appetite. False. Recent medical research, in several scientific studies, has proved that the opposite is true.

You must race the clock. False. There is no "X" time limit all men should meet at the beginning of a program for physical conditioning. It is a matter of indivdual preference. Many of the exercises must be done rapidly, but always *within your own capacity*. Quite a few must be done slowly to get the results you want.

Exercise can be "fun." False, if the object is to lose weight and become physically fit. This idea is pushed by people who urge you to take up golf, go bowling. Fine suggestions, but they have little to do with getting you in shape. The chances are you lack the time, the money or the inclination for such pursuits. No, you can't play your way back into shape.

Now that we've examined some common misconceptions about exercise, let me give you a morale-boosting fact:

Exercise is its own guarantee of success.

If you can do five push ups today, you can do eight push ups next week *with the same effort*. They follow as the night the day. You need master no technique, attain no skill. It's automatic, the God-given gift of your body.

The subject of Diet has been equally distorted and over-complicated. The experts give you charts more complex than some used by astronauts. They would limit you to a specified number of calories per day. You will even find your portions measured in grams. And those handy lists of menus for the week read like something they serve at the hospital. Yoghurt is supposed to work miracles, or seaweed, or in next month's fad perhaps finely ground coconut shells.

No matter how it's varnished, there is only one basic truth: You gain weight when your body takes in more calories in food than it expends in activity. A calorie is a measurement of energy — the amount of heat required to raise the temperature of one kilogram of water one degree centigrade.

But where does that leave you? It leaves you with a handy calorie-counter booklet which solves only half your problem. You can estimate how many calories you take in during the day, but you have no way of measuring how many calories your body is burning up. Not even your vocation can be a help in guessing this number. Another man could do your same job, eat the same food, and yet weigh 10 to 30 pounds more, or less, than you do. His motor is running at a different speed, a factor called *metabolism,* which is just as individual as you are.

So there is really only one way to find your calorie answer. Are you overweight? If your answer is "Yes," it means that your intake is greater than your outgo. You must change your eating habits *and* increase your physical activity. *Then* you will start losing weight. The number of calories you take in at the dinner table thus becomes academic.

You will notice that I have steered away from the word Diet. Actually it is a misnomer, because it has come to imply a temporary program. When I hear someone say, "I've gone on a diet," it reminds me of what I think when I hear a man say he has gone on the wagon —there is a very good chance that he will *fall off* of that wagon.

The problem of cutting down on calories is too serious for anything less than a permanent plan, something reasonable and realistic which can be undertaken without dread. This means that it won't have you walking around hungry, and it won't short you on energy. Fortunately, the science of nutrition has come a long way since the Flora Dora girls.

There are many changes in eating habits which will let you lose weight *without dieting.*

What we shall do is find the habits that suit *you.*

Three Motives

You probably have your private motives for losing weight and getting into shape. I hope you do. The exercises in this book will not demand any steely determination on your part. The principles of pound-trimming menus will not tax your capacity for self denial. But the segments of 10-15 minutes for exercise several days a week (days of your own choosing) must be consistent to be effective. Your motives are the key to this consistency.

To add to the objectives you already have, I offer three which can be resolved by even a modest program of fitness:

1. *Vanity*, the daily argument between you and your mirror, the sensual side of the healthy male. The question of vanity in any man's makeup is not whether it's there at all, but to what degree. American men are rarely forthright about an ambition to be handsome, a goal that is rather regarded as sissified or foolhardy or both. Perhaps *pride in appearance* is a phrase that will appeal to you more.

2. *Money*, not always a noble goal, is certainly rated a manly one in our society, with its accompanying payoffs in respect, comfort, power and other things happiness cannot buy. If you don't see how your financial success can get a boost from physical fitness, then you haven't given it much thought. Office fatigue is the main source of employe and customer troubles. How many times has irritableness caused you to say something harsh to an associate? How often has simple tiredness led to a whopping mistake in judgment, or in some

routine bit of work?

An oil field equipment salesman who had been on my program for six months recently said to me: "I feel like I'm taking advantage of some of these guys. They're sagging when I'm still going strong. They want to know who lit a fire under me." This man is now convinced that the fellow who doesn't tire easily will stay cheerful longer and will keep a positive approach to his work throughout the day. His conclusions are duplicates of hundreds I've heard from businessmen who've taken the trouble to get back in shape. It should not be necessary to point out how added stamina can benefit the doctor who works long hours, or the lawyer involved in lengthy negotiations.

A successful fitness program and success in business go hand-in-hand in one other respect. The strong-willed man of logical turn of mind is the first to accept a plan of exercise and weight control. And he is the same fellow who will most often have achieved a healthy bank account. That is one reason why top-ranking business executives the country over have taken to physical fitness.

3. DEATH, the ultimate spectre on creating strong motives, is a grim fellow looking over your shoulder. The most universal wish is to hang onto life's slender thread as long as possible. Let's listen to the doctors:

Dr. J. B. Wolffe, head of the Valley Forge Heart Hospital: "Regular exercise, with periods of rest, is the most important measure against the disease of the heart and premature ageing."

Dr. Paul Dudley White: "We doctors can now state from our experiences with people, both sick and well, and from a growing series of scientific researches, that keeping fit does pay rich dividends in health and longevity. As a cardiologist I have concluded from my practice of more than forty years and from current scientific investigations that keeping fit in all probability delays the onset of the major epidemic of our time, atherosclerosis."

Dr. E. L. Bortz, past president of the American Medical Association: "It begins to appear that exercise is the master conditioner for the healthy and the major therapy for the ill."

(While we are on the subject of medical opinion, let me stress that this book does not pretend to prescribe any program of exercise for men who have a history of heart ills or other major ailments. I will, however, outline in a later chapter a mild program of suggested exercises which you may submit to your physician for his approval or editing.)

Some of the scientific research to which these authorities refer, while subject to argument within the profession on technical points, seem to the layman to be as plain as the proverbial nose on your face. For instance, a 1948 survey of London bus drivers and conductors disclosed that the seatbound men, the drivers, had twice as many heart attacks as their partners, who scrambled all over the double-deck trams collecting tickets. Another study, this one by a Purdue University group, found that South Dakota farmers had half as many heart troubles as South Dakota town-dwellers.

Clearly, the energetic life is the one for the prudent man.

Now that you are armed with a few additional motives for the tough business of making a slight adjustment in your daily habits, I'll reward you with another promise: After the first few weeks of an exercise program, the sessions themselves will become the most ingrained habit you have. I'll go so far as to warn you that you'll become addicted to them. You won't feel "right" when you miss a session.

The initial purpose is all that's needed. The rest takes care of itself.

Warming Up

In this chapter and the next three chapters you will discover all of the exercises any group of men needs to know. Here are the basic body movements necessary to recondition any physique—tall, short, obese, stocky, elderly or young. There are many variations of these basic exercises, but the variations are merely icing on the cake. It may surprise you that the ones I list here are so few in number. Even if you did them all, meeting the maximum repetitions required for each, it wouldn't take you more than 25 minutes, including intermissions for rest. But you will not be called upon to do them all, or even most of them. You will find that your particular physique does not need them.

These four chapters are your tool kit. After we have demonstrated the tools, and the reasons why each is valuable for a special job, we will take a look at your requirements and then select the tools you alone need.

We'll begin with the most dangerous exercises of them all, the warm ups, which are dangerous because they are so often omitted. Athletic teams, from high school through the pros, do not frolic on the field before gametime merely for the amusement of the spectators. Partly they are sharpening their senses of timing, but mainly they are bringing their muscles awake in warning of the stresses to come. You must do the same thing before starting any exercise session.

Cornell University's study of football injuries placed a great deal of blame on the lack of warm ups before the second half kickoff. Because the following exercises are mild, do not underrate them. They perform a vital task.

1. Deep Breathing

Here is your quickest dividend: 10 deep breaths every morning. It's better, but not necessary, to take them at an open window. Really swell that rib cage to its fullest, then exhale slowly. Don't be alarmed by the green spots in front of your eyes, or a slight case of vertigo. There's nothing wrong with you except you've forgotten how to breathe.

The additional oxygen thus crammed down your throat will do wonders for your vitality. It may even bring you back from the dead on those mornings after the night before, when you don't think you can make it to noon. Our air crews in London, after a full night of wine-women-song, first made famous the recuperative powers of the oxygen tank. A few moments at the oxygen mask restored them to fighting trim before takeoff.

Precede your exercise session with the 10 deep breaths, and after you have completed the most taxing exercise on your list take 10 more. This will help restore your respiration rate to normal. It will also help swell your chest measurement. Repeat during the day, whenever you feel fatigued.

2. Jogging in Place

The ideal thing would be to prescribe a jog around your block before each exercise session, but the neighbors might think you were some kind of nut. So we'll throw out the distance requirement and keep the jog, and the time.

THE EXERCISE: Run in place, lifting your knees as high as you can without being uncomfortable about it, and keep jogging for as long as you can without being severely winded. Your goal: One minute.

Move up and down your bedroom if you wish, or a hallway, and try to keep your arms limber and let your neck muscles be slack. Come down firmly to let your heels touch the floor. This tightens the thigh muscle at the buttocks and works away the fat around the hips.

Push upwards from your toes to work your calf muscle on every stride.

This is not only a grand warm-up exercise which loosens most of the muscles about to be put in play, but it is a great relaxer, too.

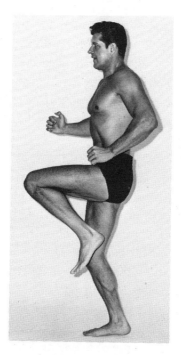

Jogging in Place

3. The Windmill

It's not necessary to touch your toes as you do this one. You might strain a muscle. This is a warm up, remember?

THE EXERCISE: Stand with your feet a little bit more than shoulder width apart. Spread your arms sideways at shoulder level. Imagine that you are holding a long broomhandle stretched across your back so that your arms will stay in direct line throughout the exercise. Now reach down with your right hand toward your left foot. Return to an erect position and reach down with your left hand toward your right foot.

The Windmill is generally supposed to be helpful in reducing the waist, and perhaps it should be, if you had time to do about 500 of them twice a day. But save your efforts for the later exercises which will really get the waistline job done. Just get loose.

4. The Tiger Stretch

The adaptation of the Tiger Stretch for humans may have been brought back to the Old World by Marco Polo, because it is certainly the oldest body conditioning exercise recorded, according to ancient Oriental documents. You have seen the big cats in the zoo, pacing up and down, then stopping every now and then to arch their torsos and hump their backs. This is the only way caged animals have of staying in physical condition.

THE EXERCISE: Support your body on hands and toes and keep your legs straight. First raise your hips as far as you can and tuck your head under with chin to chest, tightening every muscle at your command. Next, relax completely and lower your hips as close to floor as you can, bringing your head far back.

The Tiger Stretch strengthens and slenderizes the midsection and loosens up the taut muscles in your back. It is a fine "halftime warm up" in the middle of your exercise session. It is also a quick way to relax during a hard day in the business world, if you have a private office with carpeting. A couple of quick stretches will do it.

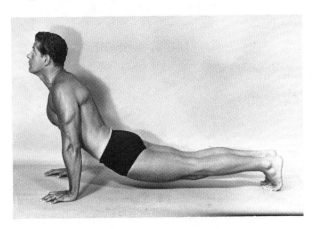

The Tiger Stretch

That Major Disaster Area — The Midsection

Nine out of ten men who are "out of shape" are out of shape where it shows the most—around the middle. The middle, in fact, is where middle age starts, beginnning in the early 20s when a fellow gives up the active life and assumes the responsibilities of a career, family, and home mortgages.

The decline of his physique can be measured from front to back, as his belt buckle keeps pushing further and further ahead of him. The older he gets, the heavier his problem. He has less time to devote to sports or the outdoor life, and now he doesn't even have the inclination.

Simple, quick, efficient exercise—no wasted motion or time—is his answer, and luckily the exercises for knocking off a bay window are the quickest and most efficient of them all.

The midsection is the key to your physique. A man who has a trim waistline will almost automatically have firm muscle tone everywhere else. That's why the *most important* exercises in this book are the ones you will find in this chapter. They are the most rewarding. But they must be performed with particular care and with an emphasis on concentration.

Do not let your mind wander while doing these exercises. Send messages to the muscles that are working. Otherwise, without realizing it, your body may bring other muscles into play and void the effect of the exercise.

18

1. Leg Raises

This one hits below the belt, where most of the trouble is. Men who are only slightly overweight first notice the added pounds just under their belt buckles—the pot belly or paunch. It is the bane of tailors the world over, and a special curse to the fellow who prefers pleatless trousers. Even active men have trouble avoiding this visitor as they near the 30s.

THE EXERCISE: Pick out a soft place to lie down. Nothing good can come of grating your backbone against a hard floor. Stay in bed, if you wish. Put your arms at your sides, palms down, and keep your feet together and legs straight. Now raise your feet 18-24 inches. Never bring your feet high enough to gain a resting interval at the peak of the raise. Now lower your feet to within three inches of the starting position. Your feet do not come to rest until the end of the exercise.

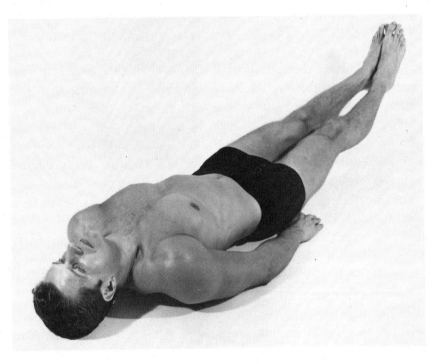

Leg Raises

2. Knee Outs

This variation of the Leg Raise will complete your attack on the lower abdomen, an area which is far harder to reduce than the upper abdomen. The Knee Out will work the same muscles in a different way, and finally will give you a natural web of strength below your belt to hold your stomach flat and trim at all times.

THE EXERCISE: From the same starting position as the Leg Raise, lift your feet together 18-24 inches and then bring your knees back toward your chest as far as you can. Now straighten your legs, still without letting your feet rest, and repeat.

These last two exercises, the Leg Raise and the Knee Out, will deceive you if you don't watch out. They are relatively easy to perform, yet they are mightily effective. *Don't* do more repetitions than your program lists for each successive day or the soreness in your lower abdomen will sideline you for a week.

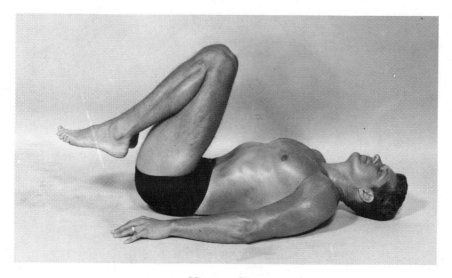

Knee Outs

3. The Sit Up

Now we hit above the belt. This is the most basic of all stomach exercises, and one of the most misunderstood. The U.S. Navy, in its World War II strength test for cadets, awarded points for each repetition up to 60. Some of the slab-bellied young men could do 150 or more before moving to the next exercise in the test. Though this might have been good for their characters, the numbers above 30—without rest intervals—didn't help their physiques at all. This is what I meant earlier in referring to *wasted motion* in exercise programs. High numbers of repetitions *tear down* the very muscles you are trying to build.

I am presuming here that all you want to do is get your waistline back to normal size. *If* you want to build a washboard-hard midsection, then you should perform sit ups in series of 25, with a minute of rest between series.

Unless the Sit Up is done properly, it is likely to result in severe muscle strains. A popular misconception is that it must be performed with hands clasped behind neck, and legs straight. This may have been quite all right for supple young men being trained to fly airplanes or

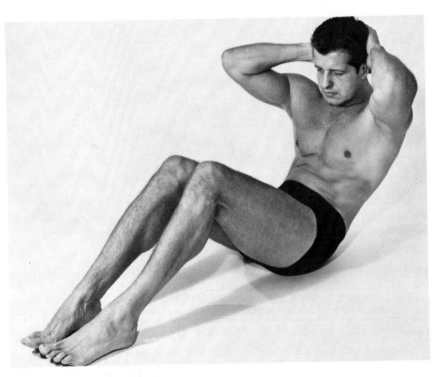

The Sit Up

ride PT boats, but it could wreak havoc on the average businessman over 25.

THE EXERCISE: Find a soft place to lie down. Stretch your arms behind or above your head. They will provide a needed boost in leverage. It will also help if someone holds your ankles in place, or if you can anchor your feet under a piece of furniture. Bring yourself to an upright sitting position first by lifting your head, then your shoulders, then your torso. Touch your fingertips to your legs as close to your feet as you comfortably can. Return to the starting position by lowering your torso, then your shoulders and finally your head.

The "roll-up" method of coming upright, instead of bringing the whole body off the floor at the same time, will ease the strain on your lower back muscles. To further ease the strain on your lower back, flex your legs slightly at the knee. Concentrate on using the stomach muscles, or the lower back will still wind up doing half the work.

As your stomach muscles gain in strength, rely less on the leverage of your arms in coming upright.

4. The Swedish Waist Reducer

How would you like to reduce your waistline by two to three inches within 30 days—through one mild exercise alone? The Swedes have the answer for you. They are one of the healthiest peoples in the world, mainly because of the natural birthrights of climate and heredity, but also because they devote so much time and thought to body conditioning. Their breathing exercise for keeping the waist in line has been in practice for centuries, and it helps account for the handsome posture of the people.

THE EXERCISE: Inhale deeply, then exhale completely. Exhalation is the secret. After all the air has been expelled from your lungs, draw in your stomach until you feel as if it's pressing against your backbone. Hold for a count of five.

That's it, simplicity itself. You can perform it several times a day —while shaving, drivng to work, at your desk, or in bed in the evening.

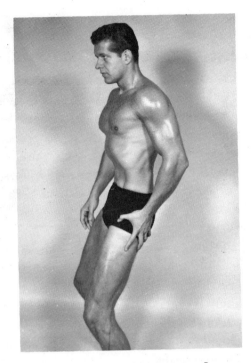

The Swedish Waist Reducer

5. Side Bends

The next time you're around someone who claims he doesn't have to do any exercise to stay trim, reach out with your thumb and fore-finger and grab the hunk of fat at his side just above the belt line. Believe me, the fat will be there. Only a concentrated exercise can hit that particular target.

THE EXERCISE: Stand erect with your left palm against your left thigh and your right palm against your right temple. Now bend to the left until your fingertips are just be-low your left knee. Return to erect position and repeat. Next switch the position of your hands and bend to the right.

These are the oblique muscles you are conditioning, the final touch to a physique that slopes naturally from shoulders to waist.

There you have the basic routines for a youthful midsection. There are dozens of other exercises which work the same area, but most are mere variations. A few can emphasize the work on a stubborn waist-line, and we will describe these special routines in a later chapter, but the majority of men can get the job done with the vital four outlined here, plus the Swedish reducer through the day.

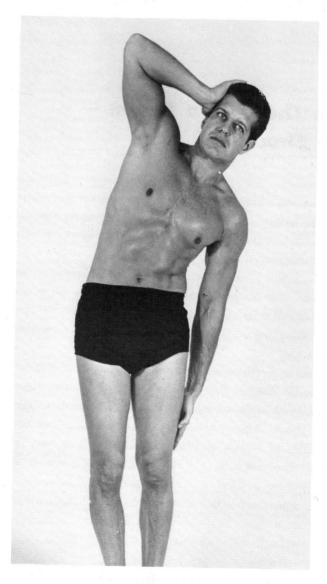

Side Bends

Where The Brawn Begins — Chest, Shoulders, Arms

A businessman's long-sleeved shirt conceals the pounds of flab that hang on his biceps and pectoral muscles, the inches of suet back of his airpits. A pudgy superstructure does not reveal itself the way a protruding stomach does.

But it is no less a matter of concern for the man who wants to feel younger and live longer. Now even the matter of concealment is growing more difficult because of the boom in outdoor living—backyard swimming pools, weekend summer homes, short-sleeved shirts for office wear.

Important as personal appearance is, the rewards in feeling fit and healthy should interest you most in getting your torso tuned up. Unlike the other deposits of fat on the body, these areas are relatively easy to re-shape. Your chest, shoulders and arms can be firmed in only a matter of weeks, and the results stick with you. Backsliders who quit an exercise program after a few months will still be able to detect the benefits to their upper body for several years.

There is something about this muscle area that stirs a man's pride in himself as a man. Perhaps it is primordial, a throwback to the days when strength was necessary to wrestle a living out of the wilderness. Or perhaps it is the tradition of doting fathers and uncles whose early request of youngsters has always been: "Show me your muscles."

1. The Push Up

This is the classic exercise for chest, shoulders and arms, an excellent three-in-one workout. With the exception of the Shoulder Dip (see below), it is the most effective routine for adding muscles quickly.

THE EXERCISE: Lie on your stomach with your feet braced against the wall or a heavy piece of furniture. Place the palms of your hands on the floor near your shoulders and push yourself up to arms' length, keeping your legs straight and your hips at all times higher than your shoulders. Now lower your body until your chin is within two or three inches of the floor and push up again.

The ideal form is to keep the body straight as a board from heels to shoulders. The coward's way out is to push his shoulders up to arms' length and then start bringing his hips up in a sway-back maneuver. If you do it this way, you are wasting your time. So begin by making sure that your hips are always higher than your shoulders. In time, as you gain strength, you will be able to lower the hips to the straight-line form.

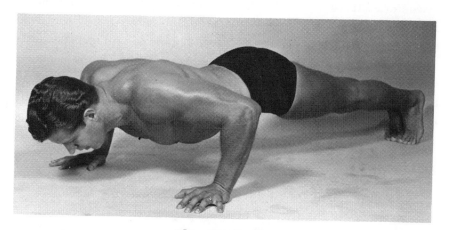

The Push Up

2. The Pull Over

Here's where you will do a double-duty chest job, expanding the rib cage and at the same time knocking off flab and building muscle.

THE EXERCISE: Lie on your back, crosswise on your bed if you prefer, and with hands together grip two books or more—a four-inch thick phone book, or two encyclopedias or three novels—any variation for the proper thickness. Keep your arms straight at all times. As you take a deep breath raise the books overhead and continue the arc until they are on the floor behind your head. Now exhale as you bring the books forward to rest on your body. Repeat, inhaling and exhaling slowly in rhythm with the movements of your arms.

The motion, not the weight of the books is the important thing here. A young fellow in training for Mr. America competition would do an entirely different exercise, with weights, to build his chest. Rember that all you are seeking is a return to normalcy.

3. The Towel Press

If you've ever been on Muscle Beach, you may have noticed that the body-beautiful devotees are never without a towel in their hands. They are forever tugging it this way and that. It is not idle habit. They are building more muscle every minute.

The ordinary bath towel is an an excellent piece of equipment in your "home gym." Used correctly, as in this exercise, it will expand the muscles at the outer edge of your shoulders, build up the forearms and also the muscles on the underside of your shoulder blades—a jackpot of benefits from one routine. But its main job is the creation of powerful triceps, the muscle which makes up two-thirds of your upper arm.

THE EXERCISE: Grasp the opposite ends of a towel in each hand and hold it behind you so that your left forearm is across the small of your back and your right arm is extended straight overhead. The palm of your left hand is facing away from your body as you grasp the towel. Now, resisting with your right arm, pull the towel downward with your left hand until your right forearm is across the back of your head and your left arm is extended straight downward. Then, resisting with your left arm, pull upward with your right until you have returned to the starting position. Next, switch position of your hands, so that the right forearm is across the small of your back and the left arm is straight overhead.

The effectiveness of the exercise will increase as your strength increases. In that way it is its own efficiency builder. A side bonus of the exercise is the help it gives your posture. The towel workout will condition your muscles to hold your shoulders back without conscious thought during the day.

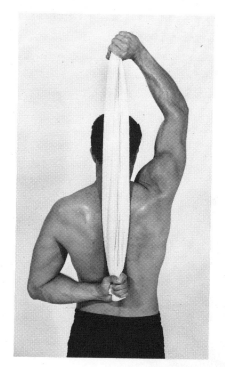 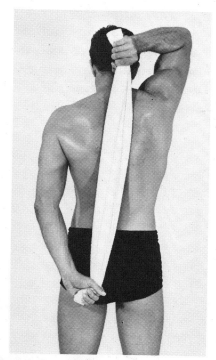

The Towel Press

4. The V Builder

The ideal of the manly physique is the sharply sloping angle of muscle from the shoulders to the waist. This is most noticeable when viewed from the back. Unless you are a stevedore on the docks, you are not likely to achieve this conformation accidentally. These muscles are the ones at the back of your armpit and just in front of the outside edge of your shoulder blades, identified in medical terms as the latissimus dorsi.

The second towel exercise is beamed directly at those muscles.

THE EXERCISE: Loop a bath towel across the edge of a door and over and under each doorknob. Grasp the ends of the towel in your two hands, like a baseball bat, and stand with your feet spread slightly more than shoulder width, flex knees. Pull the towel towards your waist slowly, then slowly let your body return to a braced position at full arms' length. Maintain a steady tug on the towel as your body moves toward and away from the door.

If a partner is available, the exercise can also be done with the other person holding one end of the towel. Because he (or she) can take a tug-of-war stance, he doesn't have to exert as much pressure as you do.

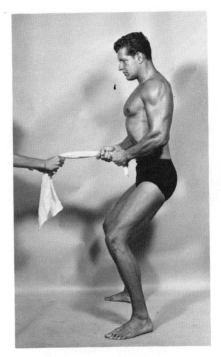

The V Builder

5. The Towel Curl

The mighty bicep is the object of this exercise, the 16-inch arm is its goal.

THE EXERCISE: In a sitting position, brace your right elbow on your right thigh near the knee. Hold both ends of a towel in your left hand and grasp the loop of the towel in your right hand, palm up. Lean forward and pull downward with your left hand while resisting with your right. Next pull upward with your right hand, resisting with your left. Your forearm should be pumping like a jack handle.

This is the old "make a muscle" motion , in spades. After finishing a session with the right arm, switch position of hands and repeat the workout with the left arm.

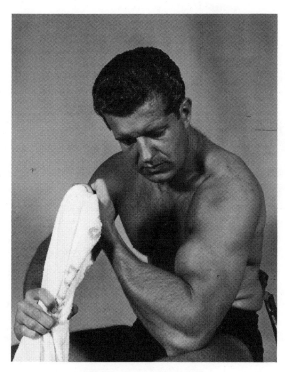

The Towel Curl

6. The Shoulder Dip

This is an extension of the Push Up. It is the most effective way to rid the upper chest of excessive flab, and to build what remains into solid muscle. It will also add muscle to widen the shoulders.

THE EXERCISE: Place two straight-back chairs face to face slightly more than shoulder width apart. Place the palms of your hands on the seats of the chairs, not far from the edge. Extend your legs behind you and keep them straight, supporting your body on the balls of your feet. Lower your torso as far as you can between the two chairs and then push yourself up to arms' length. (Once you have mastered this part of the Shoulder Dip—10 repetitions without discomfort—move on to the final stage:) Place a third chair behind you to elevate your feet. Your body will then be as horizontal as if you were doing a Push Up at floor level. Lower your torso between the chairs as before and return to arms' length position.

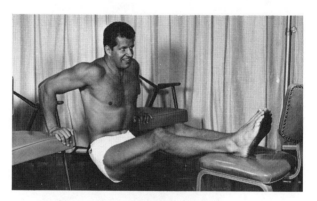

The Reverse Dip

7. The Reverse Dip

This is another V-builder, aimed at the shoulder muscles and upper back. It's also a good workout for the triceps.

THE EXERCISE: Using two facing chairs (as above). place the palms of your hands on the seats, and extend your legs in front of you, keeping them straight throughout the exercise. Now lower yourself between the chairs until your hips are only a few inches above the floor, then push up to arms' length.

You can make this Reverse Dip more effective by using a low footstool for your feet, but don't elevate them on a third chair—this presents a problem in balance which might result in severe muscle strain.

These exercises for the chest, shoulders and arms get results on two levels. They work away the fatty tissue while at the same time enlarging the muscle which is surrounded by fatty tissue. The strengthened muscle in turn helps support the fat that remains—giving you a startlingly rapid change in physical appearance.

Tired Legs—
Handicap To a Zestful Life

There are two major sources of tension for the weary businessman: 1) Taut muscles in the back and neck, 2) tired leg muscles.

Legs are the first point of deterioration in the professional athlete, most notably baseball pitchers, boxers and golfers, the latter because it affects their putting.

Here also is the origin of exhaustion for the average man. A salesman with well-conditioned legs can out-talk, out-sell and out-hustle any man in his territory. For one thing, he can keep his mind on his product, while his competitor may spend half the time looking around for a place to sit down.

The cause of all the trouble is the construction of the heel. It gives inadequate support for walking upright. The heel actually should extend further back for better balance, less reliance on the calf muscle, and more efficient performance. One of the few differences noted by anthropologists in a study of the Caucasian and Negro races is the relation of the heel to the leg. The Negro is better equipped in this regard because the heel extends for excellent leverage.

Women have had this problem solved for them by the stylishness of high-heeled shoes. Here, too, the heel of the shoe extends back of the natural heel line, allowing for a nice forward thrust on each step. A recent study of four physiologists at Springfield (Mass.) College found that the arches of the feet were improved 10 per cent by high heeled shoes. The U.S. Army, co-sponsor of the study, may decide to issue elevated combat boots to the infantry. (Cowboy boots do not apply here, because the back of the heel slopes inward.)

Aside from the conditioning angle and added strength, the following exercises also help the hefty customer melt away the extra pounds in his thighs and calves.

1. The Half Knee Bend

We'll only hit the halfway point on the famous Knee Bend exercise because it is a real knee-popper unless you were born exceptionally limber-jointed. A full knee bend risks the danger of torn knee cartilage (see below), but the half measure will still give your thigh and calf muscles plenty of pound-shedding work.

THE EXERCISE: Stand with feet about eight inches apart and place a 2- or 3-inch book under your heels. Hold your arms straight in front of you at shoulder level for balance. Keep your upper body erect as you lower your hips to the seat level of an ordinary dining room chair. You may place the chair behind you so that your rump touches the edge of it each time to remind you that you've gone far enough. Return to upright position.

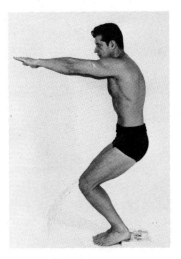

The Half Knee Bend

Concentrate on using the muscles in your calves as you straighten your legs. The concentration is focused on the calf because your thigh muscles will naturally get enough of the work. Any knee bend exercise is deceiving. You can accomplish too many of them the first effort, which will result in severe soreness, so don't be misled by your apparent prowess.

2. The Deep Knee Bend

There is only a few inches difference in degree from the Half Knee Bend above, but the difference is important. As you will note later, in the individual programs, this one is only for the muscle builder on a *weight-gaining* program.

THE EXERCISE: Take the same stance as above, book under heels, arms raised, keeping torso erect, and lower your hips *slowly.* Stop when your thighs are horizontal to the floor and return slowly to starting position.

Never allow your hips to hit bottom in the bounce-up motion that makes it easier to return upright. This excess could even tear up a teenager's knee cartilage, and in fact has led to so many knee injuries from the old squat-waddle exercise in football drills that the National Assn. of High Schools has asked that its use be banned.

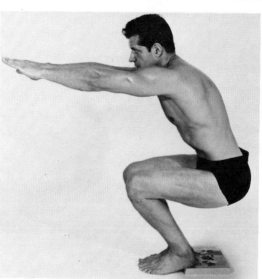

The Deep Knee Bend

3. Walking

Walking is the safest way to exercise, as witness Dr. Paul Dudley White's prescription of golf for the recuperating Dwight Eisenhower.

Walking is the vital part of every individual program for physical fitness, and probably the most neglected, even among those who become fanatical about exercise. Time is the main bugaboo. We are all so much in a hurry.

What's needed then are a few moments of thought on how to work 3-5 miles of walking into your week's routine. For instance:

—Pick a parking lot 6-8 blocks from your office. This will add a mile a day to your work week, but it could be a valuable mile. You will have to get up a bit earlier and to bed a bit earlier, a healthy combination in itself. You can use the morning walk to plan the first few hours of your day. The evening walk can give you time to unwind.

—Get to know your kids better. You may spend a lot of time *doing* things with and for your children, but how much attention do you give their more quiet problems individually? A long walk once a week, with one of them at a time, is a grand way to get close to your child. Good for him, too.

—If you're in long-walking distance of a news vendor, don't subscribe to the Sunday paper. Hike for it instead. Who knows?—your walk might even take you near a church.

—Get in the habit of walking to the store for the things your wife forgot to buy.

—Play one round of golf a week. The average golf course is 4-5 miles in length, but this suggestion is far down the list because one mile a day every day is more beneficial than five at one whack. Walking, incidentally, is the only worthwhile exercise connected with this game.

Benefits Of Your Individual Exercise Program

You know that excess weight is an invitation to ill health. But you may be surprised at the medical opinion on obesity as a factor in disease and death. You may also know of the new movement in medical science to relate *physical exercise* to the cure for obesity. But you may be surprised to learn how many old wives tales about physical exertion have been refuted by scientific study.

Let's review some of this evidence which will help you understand why an *individual* program, such as outlined for you in the succeeding chapters, is the only wise way to regain physical fitness.

Dr. Warren Guild of Harvard Medical School is one of the world's leading authorities on the relationship between physical exercise and the field of medicine. Here's what Dr. Guild says about obesity: "Obese people have a greater chance to develop heart disease, cancer, kidney illnesses, hypertension, diabetes, arthritis, and other degenerative disorders . . . There are no vaccinations or antibiotics which protect you from these illnesses. But fitness which abolishes obesity provides statistical immunization."

Fitness provides statistical immunity. But what road do you travel to achieve fitness for your own physique?

Dr. Jean Mayer has spent years of research to contradict two misconceptions about exercise which most obese people offer as an excuse for doing nothing to improve their condition. He is a Fellow of the American Assn. for the Advancement of Science, a graduate of the University of Paris, Yale University and the Sorbonne, and presently associate professor of nutrition at Harvard. In a symposium at the University of Illinois, Dr. Mayer presented a paper on Exercise and Weight Control, which refuted the two main criticisms of exercise as a means of losing weight:

1) To burn up the number of calories equal to one pound of fat, a man would have to walk for 36 hours, split wood for seven hours, or play volleyball for 11 hours.

"The implication," points out Dr. Mayer, "is that the exercise is done at one stretch. Actually, of course, the cost of splitting wood for seven hours will still be equivalent to one pound of fat even though the seven hours may not constitute one stretch. Thus, while splitting wood for seven consecutive hours would be difficult for anyone other than a Paul Bunyan, splitting wood for one half hour every day, by no means an impossible task for a healthy man, would add up to seven hours in a fortnight. If it represented a regular practice, it would, by the very reasoning of the detractors of exercise, represent the caloric equivalent of 26 pounds of body fat in a year. A half hour of handball or squash a day would be equivalent to 16 pounds a year."

2) Exercise makes you hungry. Hunger makes you eat more. Therefore, you will gain more weight because of exercise than you will lose.

An increase in activity, Dr. Mayer proved, is followed by an increase in food intake *only within a range of normal activity.*

On a program of mild exercise, beyond the range of normal activity, food intake actually *decreases.*

The other side of the coin causes all the trouble in the first place. A decrease in activity is followed by a decrease in food, again *within the range of normal activity.* That's why, in the sedentary life of the average man, the decrease in activity overtakes the decrease in food intake, resulting in obesity. Dr. Mayer points out that farmers have known this for centuries, as indicated in their practice of penning up cattle, hogs and geese for fattening. *The animals grow fat because they are denied room to exercise.*

Abstaining from food cannot be the answer by itself. "I am convinced," says Dr. Mayer, "that inactivity is the most important factor explaining the frequency of 'creeping' overweight in modern Western societies. The regulation of food intake was never designed to adapt to the highly mechanized sedentary conditions of modern life, any more than animals were made to be caged. Adaptation to these conditions without development of obesity means that either the individual will have to step up his activity *or that he will be mildly or acutely hungry all his life.*

"If stepping up activity is difficult, lifetime hunger is so much more difficult that to rely on it for weight control programs can only continue to lead to the fiascos of the past."

The relationship between food intake and exercise is the foundation of all the success I've ever had in leading men back to physical fitness. Compared to the scientific studies made by experts like Dr. Guild and Dr. Mayer, my knowledge must be defined as "empirical." That's an exact word for knowledge gained by observation and experience, rather than by principle. I have helped more than 7,000 average men to shed pounds and regain normal weight, fitness and activity through the individual programs outlined in the next chapters and through a *slight change* in their eating habits. Sir Isaac Newton, as legend has it, saw an apple drop from a tree. Sir Isaac then wanted to know why it dropped. By contrast, what interests me is that the apple drops *every time.*

I could not state the case for an individual exercise program more perfectly than does Dr. Mayer: "Strenuous exercise, on a irregular basis by untrained individuals already obese, is obviously not what is advocated here. But a reorganization of one's life to include *regular exercise adapted to one's physical potentialities* is a justified return to the wisdom of the ages."

How To Select Your Individual Program

Enroll in any of the world's exclusive and luxurious health clubs and the first order of business is taking your measurements.

But even without the measurements, the expert can tell at a glance which kind of exercise program is needed. The key to the question is the man's bone structure, plus the number of pounds overweight, and the age.

The new club member will be told that his individual exercise program will be worked out according to his vital statistics. Actually, there are only four classifications for men who are out of shape, and he will start in one of those. After the first 5-6 weeks, if a particular area refuses to respond, a special exercise for that problem will be added to his routine.

Now you can do the same. Pick out one of the four classifications which fits your physique and age, follow the detailed program prescribed for it, then after a month or so select the one or two special exercises you may need to complete the job. The following chapters deal with the four programs:

Program One—A beginner's routine, designed for men on the borderline of obesity or beyond, AND for the man over 50, regardless of how little overweight he is.

Program Two—For men of stocky build who are 25 pounds or less underweight.

Program Three—For the slender man gone to pot, the man who has a relatively thin upper body and legs, but heavy midsection and hips. Surprisingly, this is also the astronauts' program.

Program Four—for building up the thin man.

As you see, this is NOT a four-stage plan. Except for men in Program One, who move on to either Program Two or Three, depending on their bone structure, each program has its own scale of progress. And one of these programs applies specifically to you. At the end of the chapter outlining each program is a chart you can use to record your advancement. It lists the exercises and the progressive number of repetitions you are expected to achieve day by day. There are spaces for you to note how many repetitions you *do* achieve. At the bottom of the chart there is space for you to record your measurements when you begin your program, and your measurements five weeks later. Your measurements will continue to improve thereafter as you note them every month, but the initial five-week period is long enough to note real progress.

Here's how to take your measurements:

Shoulders—upper arms pressed to sides, tape circles back and chest, crossing chest at fullest point.

Chest—pass the tape under the arms this time, same level as shoulder measurement.

Waist—at the belly button.

Thighs—tape as close to groin as possible.

Arms—make a muscle and measure at peak of bicep.

Hips—circle tape at level of biggest part of buttocks.

Calf—take measurement at largest circumference.

I recommend that you buy a bathroom scale ($4-$5) and get on it at the same time every day. Your weight can vary as much as three pounds at different parts of any day. An 8 a.m. reading, for instance, will show you daily whether you are gaining or losing.

You won't discern any radical change in your weight for the first two or three weeks of your program, perhaps, but after that period you'll get a big lift out of reading the bathroom scale.

Now you are ready to proceed with your own do-it-yourself health club. The only thing you will be missing is the day-to-day encouragement and concern of an experienced trainer.

If your motives are strong enough to carry you through, you don't need him anyway.

Program One—For
Obese Or Elderly

This is the follow who is living dangerously. He is under 50, weighs over 30 pounds more than he should. Or else he is older than 50, when any excess poundage is an invitation to disaster. The weight-age ratio is a cruel one; the greater the years, the tougher the pounds.

In either case, a program of exercise should be approached with caution. The first requirement is to see your doctor—take this book with you and show him the step-by-step demands of the workout. They are mild by any standards, but are they mild enough for *you?* Only a physician can answer that question with certainty.

By failing to take an objective look at yourself, you may decide to begin Program Two or Program Three. This would be futile and possibly dangerous. You have been out of shape for years, so why expect overnight miracles now? After you have trimmed down through Program One, and I assure you that the trimming job is merely a matter of following the routine, you will be ready for *either* Program Two or Program Three, whichever fits your new physique.

This is *not* a step-up series of programs in which you are expected to advance month-by-month from Program One through Program Four. Men of any age who are 30 pounds or more overweight and men age 50 to 70 in relatively similar condition simply must be gotten into reasonable condition before tackling an earnest program like the ones that follow.

At the beginning, your main results will come from following advice in the section on eating habits, but the exercises outlined below will accelerate those results in a remarkable way.

This is *your* road to fitness:

1. *The Walking Warm-up:* Walk in place *for one minute,* lifting your knees halfway to waist level. Move your arms in unison with your legs, as you would when walking normally.

2. *Tiger Stretch:* Support your body on hands and toes and keep your legs straight. First raise your hips as far as you can and tuck your head under with chin to chest. Next, relax completely and lower your hips as close to floor as you can, bringing your head far back. *Begin with three repetitions, increase gradually to 12.*

3. *One-Leg Raise:* Lie on back, bring your right knee toward chest. Keep left leg straight; lift it 18-24 inches, then lower it within three inches of starting point. Next, bring your left knee toward chest and repeat exercise with right leg. *Begin with three, each leg, increase to 12.*

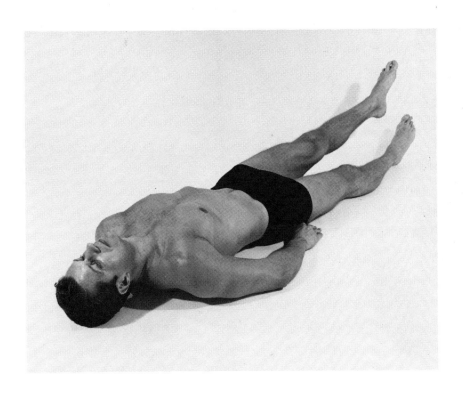

One-Leg Raise

4. *Pull-Over:* Lie on your back and with hands together grip two or three books at arms' length. Inhale deeply and raise books overhead until they touch the floor behind you. Exhale as you bring books back to starting position. *Begin with five, increase to 25.*

(REST FOR ONE MINUTE.)

5. *Half Knee Bend:* Stand with feet about eight inches apart and place a two- or three-inch book under your heels. Hold arms straight in front of you at shoulder level. Keep your body erect as you lower hips to seat level of straight chair. Then return to upright position. *Begin with three, increase to 12.*

6. *The Swedish Waist Reducer:* Take a deep breath and exhale completely. Before next breath, draw stomach in as far as you can, hold it there for count of five. Begin with two, four times daily. After five days increase to four sets of *three* repetitions. *Increase repetitions to 10.*

7. *Walking:* This is more important to your program than it is for other men who are able to tackle strenuous exercises. *One mile daily.*

Mark your progress on the following chart. Don't force yourself to hit the desired repetitions in the required number of days unless you feel comfortable doing them. Follow the program five days a week, taking Saturday and Sunday off except for your walking requirements. (See Point 7, above.)

Within six weeks you will see that you are progressing to the next step for full conditioning, and shortly after that you will be close enough to your normal weight to begin more strenuous exercises.

THE BEGINNER'S CHART

Exercise	M	T	W	T	F	M	T	W	T	F	M	T	W	T	F	M	T	W	T	F	M	T	W	T	F
Walk in Place	One Minute																								
Tiger Stretch	3	4	5	5	5	6	6	6	7	7	7	7	8	8	9	9	9	10	10	10	11	11	11	12	12
One-Leg Raise	3	4	5	5	5	6	6	6	7	7	7	7	8	8	9	9	9	10	10	10	11	11	11	12	12
Pull Over	5	6	7	8	9	10	11	12	13	14	14	14	15	16	18	19	20	21	22	23	24	25	25	25	25
Half Knee Bend	3	4	5	5	5	6	6	6	7	7	7	7	8	8	9	9	9	10	10	10	11	11	11	12	12
Swedish Reducer			4 sets 2 daily					4-3s					4-4s					4-5s					2-10s + 2-5s		
Walking	One Mile Daily																								

Measurements At Start Of Program

Shoulders_____ Chest_____ Arms_____

Waist_____ Hips_____ Thighs_____

Calf_____ Weight_____

Measurements After Five Weeks

Shoulders_____ Chest_____ Arms_____

Waist_____ Hips_____ Thighs_____

Calf_____ Weight_____

Program Two—For
The Stocky Man

Are you short-waisted and thick-legged? Has Nature and the soft life spread corpulence with equal disfavor to your upper body as well as your midsection? Are you between 10 and 30 pounds overweight? Then this is your chapter. Program Two is designed specifically for you.

You were originally blessed with a good set of shoulders, an expansive rib cage, and a strong wide-set bone structure in the hips. Fully muscled and trimmed down to your normal weight, you would still have a relatively thick waist, but it would all add up to a powerful, admirable physique.

The stocky man—who may not be short at all, and at six feet may carry a normal weight of 195, or 40 pounds more than a fellow of slight bone structure—has outstanding potential for performing strenuous exercise with less effort than his smaller or taller brothers.

But the stocky man is also in constant danger of ballooning way out of shape. His frame is an open invitation to an added five pounds a year.

The goal of this individualized exercise program is 1) to shed the excess fat on his upper body, his legs and his thighs, while at the same time firming the fine muscle structure that remains in those areas; 2) to trim away the adipose condition of his waistline and strengthen the muscles to support the natural weight which will always remain there.

The end result will be the accepted ideal of the American male physique: A normal chest measurement 10 inches more than the waist measurement.

The program is charted for five weeks of five days each, Monday through Friday, an interval in which you should be able to reach the maximum number of repetitions required for each exercise. If you have not hit the maximum on one or two exercises within the five weeks keep up the Monday-Friday schedule until you do. Then, if you have followed the advice on changed eating habits, you may cut back to a three-day week and keep that as your regular routine. I would suggest a Monday-Wednesday-Friday schedule for the man who has the weekend off, or any three-day combination within the work week, with a day's rest between workouts.

The first five weeks are the key to your whole future. They are enough to establish a routine of habit, and a conditioning of the body, which will practically compel you to keep on with the three-day week. You will then be spoiled by the refreshing qualities of the workouts, and your body will demand attention from you.

Don't get carried away by your enthusiasm and try to start this program in the middle of the week. Do one or two repetitions of the exercises as you read them, so you'll understand them completely. Then wait until you can begin five consecutive days of work. Let the required number of repetitions be a guide, not an unbreakable law. If you feel distress after completing eight Push Ups, stay at eight for a few days before increasing to nine.

Don't neglect the intervals between exercises which require 10 deep breaths. This gives your body time to recover from the previous exercise and will help you succeed on the next one. In fact, it's not at all necessary that these exercises be done in an uninterrupted stretch. If you choose to plan your exercise sessions for the mornings, you may work them into your normal routine—brush your teeth, say, after the Sit Ups; shave after the Knee Bends; and shower after the Push Ups. Whichever way you choose to do them, the exercises will not add more than 10-15 minutes to your morning preparations. They will require considerably less time than that at the beginning, when the repetitions are fewest.

Don't fear that you're losing any of the value of the program if you do the exercises in late morning, mid-afternoon or even at night. The time of day is irrelevant.

Here is *your* road to physical fitness:

Warm Up: Jog in place for *one minute.* Lift knees high. Let muscles in arms and neck and shoulders go slack.

Spread feet just beyond shoulder width, arms outstretched from shoulders. Keep arms in direct line as you reach toward left foot with right hand, come erect, then reach toward right foot with left hand. *Begin with five, increase to 25, each side.*

1. *The Sit Up:* Lie on back with arms together and outstretched above you. Have feet anchored at ankles. Come to sitting position by first lifting head, then shoulders, then torso. Extend arms toward toes. Recline slowly. *Begin with five, go to 25.*

2. *Side Bend:* Stand erect, left arm along side, palm of right hand against right temple. Bend to the left until fingertips reach knee or below. Switch position of hands and bend right. *Begin with five, increase to 25, each side.*

(Take 10 Deep Breaths.)

3. *Leg Raises:* Lie on back, arms at sides, plams to floor. Keep legs straight, raise them together 18-24 inches, then lower to within three inches of starting position. *Begin with five, increase to 25.*

4. *Pull Over:* Lie on your back and with hands together grip two or three books at arms' length. Inhale deeply and raise books overhead until they touch the floor behind you. Exhale as you bring books back to starting position. *Begin with 10, increase to 30.*

5. *Half Knee Bends:* Stand with feet about eight inches apart and place a two- or three-inch book under your heels. Hold arms straight in front of you at shoulder level. Keep your body erect as you lower hips to seat level of straight chair. Then return to upright position. Perform rapidly. *Begin with five, increase to 25.*

6. *Tiger Stretch:* Support your body on hands and toes and keep your legs straight. First raise hips as far as you can and tuck your head under with chin to chest. Next, relax completely and lower hips as close to floor as you can, bringing head far back. *Begin with five, increase to 25.*

7. *Push Ups:* Lie on your stomach with feet braced against a wall or heavy piece of furniture. Place the palms of your hands on the floor near your shoulders and push up to arms' length, keeping legs straight and hips slightly higher than shoulders. Next, lower your body until chin is within two or three inches of floor and push up again. *Begin with five, increase to 20.*

8. *Walking:* Minimum five miles a week.

PROGRAM TWO
CHART FOR THE STOCKY MAN

Exercise	M	T	W	T	F	M	T–F	M	T–F	M	T–F	M	T–F
Jogging Windmill (One Minute)	5	6	7	8	9	10	11 - 14	15	16 - 19	20	21 - 24	25	25 - 25
Side Bends	5	6	7	8	9	10	11 - 14	15	16 - 19	20	21 - 24	25	25 - 25
Sit Ups	5	6	7	8	9	10	11 - 14	15	16 - 19	20	21 - 24	25	25 - 25
Leg Raises	5	6	7	8	9	10	11 - 14	15	16 - 19	20	21 - 24	25	25 - 25
Pull Overs	10	11 - 14				15	16 - 19	20	21 - 24	25	26 - 29	30	30 - 30
Half Knee Bends	5	6	7	8	9	10	11 - 14	15	16 - 19	20	21 - 24	25	25 - 25
Tiger Stretch	5	6	7	8	9	10	11 - 14	15	16 - 19	20	21 - 24	25	25 - 25
Push Ups	5	6	7	8	9	10	11 - 14	15	16 - 19	20	21 - 24	25	25 - 25

Measurements At Start Of Program

Shoulders _____ Chest _____ Arms _____
Waist _____ Hips _____ Thighs _____
Calf _____ Weight _____

Measurements After Five Weeks

Shoulders _____ Chest _____ Arms _____
Waist _____ Hips _____ Thighs _____
Calf _____ Weight _____

Program Three—For Pear Shapes And Astronauts

This is the case of the thin man gone to seed, the fellow of slight build who got massive around the middle. Or the tall hombre who has put all his weight in the basement.

The pear-shaped physique requires a double prescription of conditioning. The chest, shoulders, arms and legs must be built up. The hips and midsection must be trimmed down. You will be pleased to learn that the remedy does not, however, require double effort.

What it does require is a double dose of honesty. You may be reluctant to admit that you belong in this sad category. A face saving factor is that you are about to begin the program of fitness which is followed by the astronauts in Houston.

How is this for a conversation topper?—"Yes, I've been working out at home. Doing the same set of exercises as Alan Shepard and those fellows going to the moon." You will be telling the truth, because the Pear Shape's fitness plan is an all-around body conditioning routine which also happens to be ideal for a man already in shape. Besides Shepard, I have prescribed this program for the new set of astronauts: Charley Conrad, Frank Borman, James McDivitt, Jim Lovell and Tom Stafford.

So Mr. Pear Shape is in select company.

He has another thing going for him—his appearance is deceiving.

He *seems* to be a great deal more overweight than he actually is. He has a fat man's profile, but not the fat man's problems. The job is to redistribute the weight as much as it is to lose it.

When his midsection and hips are brought down to proportion with the rest of him, he is suddenly a slender, well-muscled fellow. It is much easier for him to lose surplus pounds because he is not cursed with a Fat Man's metabolism.

The mild increase in physical activity outlined below will call for a two-way program of conditioning. You must vary the speed of the exercises. The muscle builders are performed in a slow, deliberate rhythm; the waist trimmers are repeated as fast as possible. Slow to build muscle. Fast to melt away pounds.

A further difference is the number of sessions and how they are spread. A day of rest is needed between sessions of muscle building to give the muscles time to recuperate and feed themselves. On a Monday-through-Friday schedule, skip the muscle builders on Tuesdays and Thursdays. On Monday, Wednesday and Friday do them *before* you do the waist trimmers.

Here is *your* road to physical fitness:

Warm Up: Jog in place for *one minute.* Lift knees waist high as you jog.

Spread feet just beyond shoulder width, arms outstretched from shoulders. Keep arms in direct line as you reach toward left foot with right hand, come erect, then reach toward right foot with left hand. *Begin with five, increase to 25.*

1. *V Builder:* Loop a bath towel across the edge of a door and over and under each doorknob. Grasp the ends of the towel in your two hands, like a baseball bat, and stand with your feet spread slightly more than shoulder width, knees flexed. Pull the towel towards your waist slowly, then slowly let your body return to a braced position at full arms' length. Maintain a steady tug on the towel as your body moves toward and away from the door. *Begin with five, increase to 10.*

2. *Towel Press:* Grasp the opposite ends of a towel in each hand and hold it behind you so that your left forearm is across the small of your back and your right arm is extended straight overhead. The

palm of your left hand is facing away from your body as you grasp the towel. Resisting with your right arm, pull towel downward until the right forearm is across the back of your neck and left arm is fully extended. Next, resisting with left hand, pull upward to return to starting position. Switch hands and repeat exercise. *Begin with five, increase to 10.*

3. *Pull Over:* Lie on your back and with hands together grip two or three books at arms' length. Inhale deeply and raise books over head until they touch floor behind you. Exhale as you bring books back to starting position. *Begin with 10, increase to 30.*

4. *Half Knee Bends:* Stand with feet about eight inches apart and place two- or three-inch book under your heels. Hold your arms straight in front of you at shoulder level. Keep your torso erect as you lower hips to seat level of ordinary straight chair. Return to upright position. *Begin with five, increase to 10.*

5. *Shoulder Dip:* Place two straight-back chairs face to face slightly more than shoulder width apart. Place palms on the seats of the chairs. Extend legs behind you and keep them straight, supporting your body on the balls of your feet. Lower torso between the two chairs almost to the floor and then push yourself up to arms' length. After reaching goal of 10 repetitions, place a third chair behind you and elevate your feet. Lower your body between chairs and push up as before. *Increase to a goal of 10 repetitions.*

6. *Reverse Dip:* Use two facing straight chairs (as above) and place the palms of your hands on the seats. Extend your legs in front of you and keep them straight. Lower yourself between the chairs until your hips are within a few inches of the floor, then push up with arms to starting position. *Begin with five, increase by one per session to 10.*

THE WAIST TRIMMERS — 5 DAYS A WEEK
(For Five Weeks)

1. *Sit Ups:* Lie on your back, stretch your arms above or behind your head and anchor your feet under a heavy piece of furniture. Bring yourself to an upright position first by lifting your head, then your shoulders, then your torso. Touch your fingertips as close to your feet as you can. Return to starting position by lowering your torso, then your shoulders and finally your head. *Begin with five,*

increase daily to 25.

2. *Side Bends:* Stand erect with your left palm against your left thigh and your right palm against your right temple. Bend to the left until your fingertips are just below your left knee. Return to erect position and repeat. Next switch position of hands and bend to the right. *Begin with five, increase to 25, each side.*

3. *Knee Outs:* Lie on your back, arms at sides, legs straight. Lift your feet together 18-24 inches without bending knees, then bring knees back toward chest as far as you can. Next straighten your legs without letting feet touch floor and repeat. *Begin with five, increase to 25.*

Walking: A Minimum of five miles a week.

*   *   *   *

After five weeks of the combined program, muscle builders and weight trimmers, you will have made enough progress to cut the waist trimming sessions to three times a week.

PROGRAM THREE
CHART FOR THE THIN-FAT MAN

Exercise	One Minute	M T W T F	M T W T F	M T W T F	M T W T F	M T W T F
Jog Windmill	One Minute	5 6 7 8 9	10 11 - 14	15 16 - 19	20 21 - 24	25 25 - 25
The V Builder		5 6 7 8 9	10			10
Towel Press		5 6 7 8 9	10			10
Pull Over		10 11 12-14	15 16 17-19	20 21 - 24	25 26 - 29	30 30 - 30
Half Knee Bends		5 6 7 8 9	10			10
Shoulder Dip (In 2 Stages)		5 6 7 8 9	10 10 10 5 6	7 8 9 10		10
Reverse Dip		5 6 7 8 9	10			10
Sit Ups		5 6 7 8 9	10 11 - 14	15 16 - 19	20 21 - 24	25 25 - 25
Leg Raises		5 6 7 8 9	10 11 - 14	15 16 - 19	20 21 - 24	25 25 - 25
Side Bends		5 6 7 8 9	10 11 - 14	15 16 - 19	20 21 - 24	25 25 - 25
Knee Outs		5 6 7 8 9	10 11 - 14	15 16 - 19	20 21 - 24	25 25 - 25

Measurements At Start Of Program

Shoulders____Chest____Arms____

Waist____Hips____Thighs____

Calf____Weight____

Measurements After Five Weeks

Shoulders____Chest____Arms____

Waist____Hips____Thighs____

Calf____Weight____

Program Four–For
The Thin Man

Remember the skinny guy in the ads in the comic pages? Skinny went to the beach, where a big bruiser kicked sand in his face and walked off with his girl. The last panel advised him to drink Ovaltine. At other times Skinny was told to send away for a Charles Atlas course in muscle building. ("I was a 98-pound weakling.")

Both remedies have merit, but the curse of the Thin Man today is not as severe as it once was. He has the example of Frank Sinatra and Sexy Rexy Harrison to guide him on essays into romance. And he has the constant envy of his fat brothers: "If I ate like that, I would weigh 300 pounds."

The dire consequences of being thin today are more subtle, much more complex. The Thin Man's personality and emotional stability—nerve-wracked and high-strung—are dictated by his poor physical condition. Consider how moments of tiredness affect him. Low stamina leaves him with a feeling of lassitude in his body, but his motor is still running. His inherent metabolism, the high rate with which his system burns up fat, goes on as before. So there he sits: too tired to move, too revved up to stay still. There's got to be an explosion. And it usually shows in irritableness, irrational impulse, and sometimes in stomach ulcers.

On top of it all, maybe he *does* want to look like Charles Atlas.

A great deal of his problems will be solved by a change in eating habits, as we shall see later in a special chapter on weight-gaining. But simultaneously he will have to follow an exercise program, or else he will wind up in the same boat with Mr. Pear Shape.

The thin man's routine of exercises requires longer to complete (about 15 minutes) because it cannot be hurried. All the exercises must be performed with deliberation, and in a slow rhythmic fashion. On the other hand, Thin Man requires fewer days in the week, because his sessions must be spaced with a day of rest in between. This interval gives the muscles time to recuperate and grow between workouts.

It will probably be six to eight weeks before the difference can be noted on a tape measure, but the change will be evident almost from the beginning, as noted in the mirror. The sagging muscles of the chest and arms will take new form right away, as a prelude to growing larger. And the factor of pure stamina, reflected in a new zest for life, will be apparent from the start.

Thin Man, this is *your* road to fitness:

The Warm Up: Jog in place, lift your knees high, come down on your feet in a toe-and-heel landing, push off from the heel and then the toe to get thigh and calf muscles into action. *Continue for one minute.*

1. *Tiger Stretch:* Support your body on hands and toes and keep your legs straight. First raise your hips as far as you can and tuck your head under with chin to chest. Next relax completely and lower your hips toward floor and bring your head far back. *Begin with five, increase to 15.*

2. *V Builder:* Loop a bath towel across the edge of a door and over and under each doorknob. Grasp the end of the towel in your two hands, like a baseball bat, and stand with your feet spread slightly more than shoulder width, knees flexed. With arms extended you should be leaning at a definite angle away from the door edge. Now pull the towel as if to bring it straight toward your waist, resisting with the lean of your body as it is slowly pulled toward upright position. Then slowly let your body return to starting position at full arms' length. Maintain a steady tug on the towel as your body moves

toward and away from the door. *Begin with five, increase to 10.*

3. *Pull Over:* Lie on your back and with hands together grip two books or more—a four inch thick phone book, or two encyclopedias or three novels—any variation for the proper thickness. Keep your arms straight. As you take a deep breath raise the books overhead and continue the arc until they are on the floor behind you. Now exhale as you bring the books forward to rest on your body. Repeat, inhaling and exhaling slowly in rhythm with the movements of your arms. *Begin with five, increase one a day to a total of 10.*

4. *Deep Knee Bend:* Stand erect with arms extended in front of you for balance, and with a two- or three-inch book placed under the heels. Now lower your hips slowly until your thighs are horizontal to the floor, and return to starting position. *Begin with five, increase to 10.* (After five weeks, do three sets of 10.)

5. *Towel Curl:* In sitting position, brace your right elbow on your right thigh near the knee. Hold both ends of a towel in your left hand and grasp the loop of the towel in your right hand, palm up. Lean forward and pull downward with your left hand while resisting with your right. Next pull upward with your right hand, resisting with your left. Your forearm should be pumping like a jack handle. *Begin with five, each arm, increase to 10.*

6. *Shoulder Dip:* Place two straight-back chairs face to face slightly more than shoulder-width apart. Place palms on chair seats, extend legs behind you and keep them straight, support your body on the balls of your feet. Lower torso between the two chairs as far as you can and then push yourself up to arms' length. *Begin with five (or as many as you can do) and increase to 10.* After three sessions at 10, use a third chair to support your feet and begin at five again, working up to 10. After five weeks, do three sets of 10.

7. *The Reverse Dip:* Use two facing straight chairs (as above) and place palms on chair seats. Extend legs in *front* of you and support body on heels. Lower yourself between chairs as if you were going to sit on the floor, keeping legs straight. Within a few inches of floor push up with arms to starting position. *Begin with five, increase to 10.* (After five weeks, do three sets of 10, with 30-second rest periods between sets.)

PROGRAM FOUR
CHART FOR THE THIN MAN

Exercise	M T W T F (One Minute)	M T W T F	M T W T F	M T W T F	M T W T F	M T W T F
Jogging	5 6 7 8 9	10 11 12 13 14 15				15
Tiger Stretch	5 6 7 8 9	10				10
The V Builder	5 6 7 8 9	10				10
Pull Over	5 6 7 8 9	10				10
Deep Knee Bend	5 6 7 8 9	10				10
Towel Curl	5 6 7 8 9	10				10
Shoulder Dip	5 6 7 8 9	10				10
Reverse Dip	5 6 7 8 9	10				10

MEASUREMENTS AT START

Shoulders _____ Chest _____ Arms _____

Waist _____ Hips _____ Thighs _____

Calf _____ Weight _____

MEASUREMENTS AFTER FIVE WEEKS

Shoulders _____ Chest _____ Arms _____

Waist _____ Hips _____ Thighs _____

Calf _____ Weight _____

How To Keep The Shape You've Earned

All right, have I missed anyone along those four roads to fitness? Yes, I have. There is one man left, the trim fellow at his natural weight who wants to stay trim. Perhaps he feels a paunch coming on. Aside from improvements in physique, this man needs the physiological benefits of exercise, too, as indicated by recent evidence being uncovered in the studies of heart disease and cholesterol.

This Mr. Trim Man is also *you* — you, that is, after you have worked yourself into shape via one of the preceding programs. You have earned the right to stay in shape, which is a far much simpler thing than getting there.

The trim man's regimen will be yours to follow daily as a way of life. The fitness routines of the previous chapters were not meant for perpetual use. They are a guide back to normalcy.

The answer at this point is the Perfect Hundred—four basic exercises of 25 repetitions each. This daily hundred will keep your muscles toned up, your midsection flattened down, your stamina high and your personality smooth. They will be your personal barometer of physical fitness: Whenever you have difficulty performing them at your usual speed, you will know that you are backsliding down the fitness scale.

A big factor is that the Perfect Hundred will not demand much of your time, because the main requirements of the exercises call for speed in execution. A time limit of 3½ minutes, just 210 seconds, is your goal.

Warm Up: Jog in place for 45 seconds, lifting knees high and stepping fast. If you don't want to time yourself, count 60 strides.

25 Push Ups: Start with this one because it is the most taxing and you want to be fresh when you sail into it. Keep body line straight as you support body on palms and balls of your feet, lowering to within three inches of floor and pushing up to arms' length rapidly.

25 Sit Ups: Have your feet firmly anchored and your knees flexed slightly. From starting position on your back, you should come upright in a roll-up motion, head first, then shoulders, then torso, and touch your toes with your fingertips.

25 Knee Bends: Do these in a hurry, too, but be sure not to bounce down to your heels. Stop downward motion when thighs are horizontal to floor. Also, straighten legs completely at the finish of each repetition.

25 Leg Raises: From starting position on your back, arms at sides, keep legs straight as you move them up and down together from 18-24 inches to three feet at peak of lift.

The Finish: End the session with 45 seconds jogging in place, as in warm up.

Your total elapsed time at the beginning should be about five minutes. The lineup may appear to be rigorous, but for a man in good condition it isn't. And it's a routine he can stay with for years, on up through his 60s. The jogging sessions will strengthen the areas in your legs and hips which the four exercises neglect. Two of the four are aimed at your midsection, because that's where your years tend to catch up with you.

In a few short weeks, you'll do the session in two minutes!

Calf Lift

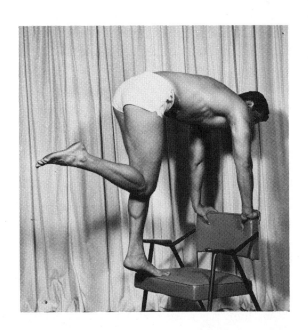

Shoulder Dip

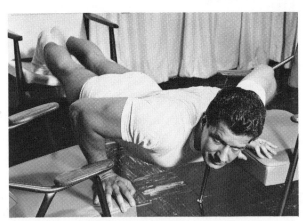

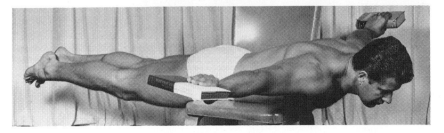

Book Swim

63

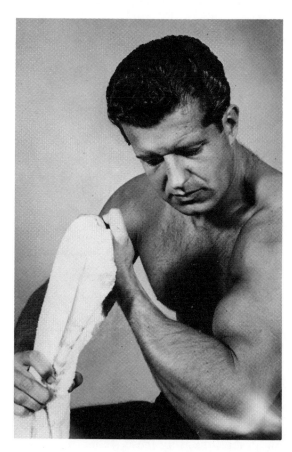

Towel Curl

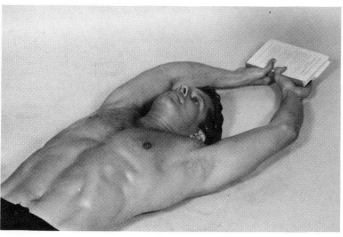

Pull Over

Special Exercises—To Each His Own

The fitness programs prescribed for the four main types of physiques should get the job done for a majority of men. There is a minority, however, who have hell's own time solving their problems.

A long-waisted fellow may have large chunks of fat on the backs of his thighs, and when he says he can feel his food hit bottom, he is speaking literally. Or another man may have excessive rolls of fat at his waistline along his sides. The basic exercises I have emphasized up to now may be too slow in melting away these stubborn areas.

You can detect your own trouble spots easily. After five weeks on the basic exercises in your program, you will note the areas where you are not getting results. Pick out one of the remedies which follow and add it to your routine.

These supplemental exercises are also useful in adding variety to your regular program. If you are a man who abhors day-after-day routines of any kind, sub a few of these boosters into your lineup from week to week.

Chacun à son goût is the French phrase for "to each his own." Pick out the chacun you dig the most.

1. Calves And Thighs

The Calf Lift: Face a straight chair, put the ball of your right foot on the edge of the seat and grasp the chairback with both hands.

Step up so that your entire body is supported by the right foot. Now arch your foot to raise the right heel as far as you can. Next lower it as far as you can. Start with five on each foot and increase by one per session.

Sissy Squats: A rugged variance of the half knee bend. Muscle-men gave it the sissy tag because it is done without weights. The secret is to lean backward as far as you can without losing balance and bend your knees forward, hand on hips. The increased leverage puts tremendous demands on your thigh muscles. Do these rapidly, beginning with five and increasing one per session to 10. At that point start doing them in three sets of 10, with a brief rest between sets.

Thigh Thrust: Lie on your back with knees drawn up so that your feet are flat on the floor (or bed). Arms are at your sides, palms down. Concentrating on the use of your thigh muscles lift your hips as high as you can, then lower to within an inch of original position and lift again. Start with five, work up to three sets of 10.

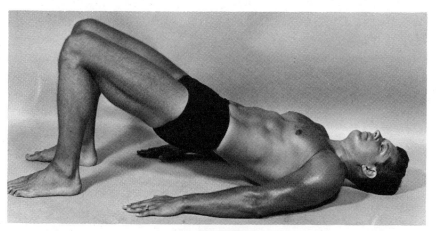

Thigh Thrust

2. The Hips

The Hip Roll: Lie on your back (the floor is recommended for this one, softened by a doubled blanket to prevent bruising) with your arms outstretched and palms down. Keeping your legs straight, cross your right leg over your left as far as you can and touch your right toe to the floor. Return to starting position and cross your left leg

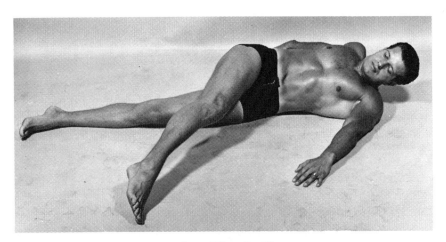

The Hip Roll

over the right. Do five crossovers with each leg at the start, and work up to three sets of 10.

The Kickaway: Face the back of a straight chair and hold onto the top with both hands. Rise up on the ball of your right foot and lift the left leg as far up in back of you as you can without bending the knee. Next stand on the ball of your left foot and lift the right leg the same way. Start with five on each leg and work up to three sets of 10.

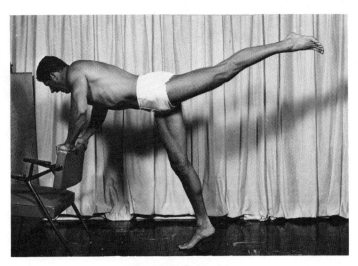

The Kickaway

3. Chest And Shoulders

The Book Swim: Balance yourself on your stomach across an armless straightback chair. If this is too neat a trick for you, lie crosswise on the bed so that your chest and shoulders are extended over the edge. Grasp two books in each hand with arms outstretched straight in front of you. Now move your arms to the side, as in a breaststroke swimming motion. This one can be tough, so start with three and increase one per session to a goal of 20.

4. The Waistline

The Twist: The big difference between this version and that crazy dance is that here you move the hips as little as possible. Rigidity of the hips, in fact, is essential for best results. Feet slightly spread, arms outstretched as if holding a broomstick across the back of your neck, turn upper torso until your hands are fore and aft of you, at right angle to your starting position. Keep the hips forward at all times. Now turn the other way. Do the exercise on a count of 1-2 3 for one minute. Start slowly the first few times you try it, gradually increasing the number of turns you do in the 60-second period.

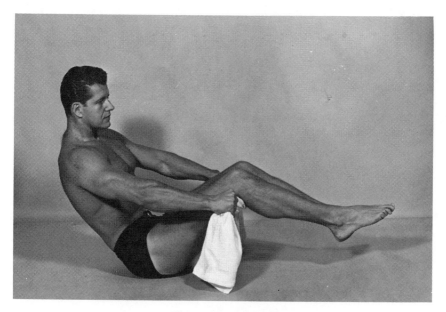

The Towel Lift

The Towel Lift: This is a *rugged* workout for the lower abdomen. Sit on the floor or bed, holding the ends of a towel with arms straight in front of you. Keeping your feet together and your body erect, lift feet just barely off the floor, draw your knees toward you and then extend your legs across the top of the towel. Now draw your knees back again and slowly return your legs to the starting position. Repeat immediately without pausing to rest. At the beginning you will have trouble keeping your upper body erect and maintaining your balance. Start with three and increase by one daily to a goal of 10.

Before You Change
The Menu

Remember I promised you that it is easy to lose weight. The promise held two requirements. First, you had to increase the amount of calories your body uses for energy. Your individual exercise program takes care of that. Second, you had to decrease the amount of calories you shovel in at the dinner table.

That sounds like the hard part. But it isn't. You've already made it half as difficult by increasing your physical activity. Before we start talking calories, let's see how we can make it even easier.

Few of us have the will power to follow a strictly regimented diet, unless, of course, the doctor has given us six months to live. If that's your case, you're in better hands than mine. What we really need is a sensible system of food intake which we can follow forever. Not a "diet" at all.

And if there is going to be any self sacrifice involved, a dismal prospect, we want to make sure that it pays off. To this end, after years of prescribing menus for weight control, I have arrived at a general set of rules on eating. Most of them are as old as common sense, but I have found that plain common sense often vanishes when the mashed potatoes hit the table.

If these principles seem like a radical change for you, don't be discouraged. On the contrary, this may mean that most of your trouble is not what you eat, but *how* and *when*.

These are my 10 commandments of good eating:

1. *Don't skimp breakfast.* Here's your best opportunity to store up a lot of nourishment without adding any fat to your goodly supply, so don't pass it up. After a good night's rest your body is ready to wear off the effects of food at full speed.

2. *Load Up At Mid-Day.* Your noon meal should be the big meal of your day, which is a neat trick I'll agree for the working man. If you can afford the added expenditure of time or money, or both, don't hesitate. Go home for lunch, if possible. Or find a restaurant that serves something besides sandwiches. You have a hard-working afternoon ahead of you to burn up the groceries.

3. *The Three-Hour Fast.* If Gandhi could do it for weeks, you can make it the last three hours before bedtime. Avoid TV programs which have food commercials. Put a time lock on your refrigerator. Anything. But eat supper at least three hours before you hit the sack, and nothing afterward, until the next morning.

4. *Don't skip a meal.* Oho, you like this one? Aside from the wear and tear on your nervous system, skipping a meal (lunch, for instance) may actually cause you to gain weight. The explanation of this has to do with your metabolism. Meanwhile, believe me, the sacrifice of one of your three squares costs you more than its worth.

5. *Don't eat between meals.* There are two reasons, only one of which is obvious: the added calories. The second is equally important. Between-meal snacks cut down your enjoyment of the food you will eat at the regular hour.

6. *Don't deny your sweet tooth.* This is another good one. Most diets fail because they ask you to give up sweets completely. *Honey* is the answer. Raw, natural honey. Use it as a sweetener—in coffee, on toast, spread over fresh fruits and some salads. Besides having less caloric count than sugar, it is more easily released in energy through your body. Parry O'Brien, the Olympic shotput champion, popularized honey among trackmen as a quick energizer. Also, it's a lazy man's food. The bee has already digested it for you.

7. *Avoid alcohol.* Joe E. Lewis claims he sees a lot more old drunks around than old doctors. Nevertheless, cut down to a minimum if you want to start losing weight. At least omit that *second* drink before dinner. Think of it this way: That drink is cheating you out of a lot of meat and potatoes. And it gives you the false notion you can eat a horse. After you're back to normal weight, you can resume toping in moderation. Red Bordeaux with your meals will be the best bet.

8. *Don't omit liquids.* Drink at least six glasses of water or natural fruit juices every day. Mainly this is a stipulation of good health. It may also kid your stomach into thinking there's the same amount of traffic as there used to be.

9. *Listen to Grandma.* Remember how parents in the old days used to say, "Don't bolt your food?" Then there was the period when psychologists believed if you insisted that a kid chew his food better he might get up from the table and go rob a bank. Anyway, Grandma was right, even though you thought she was only concerned with your manners. The greatest single secret for losing weight is the careful mastication of food before it goes down the pipe. The reason is simple. Food is more *filling* when you chew it thoroughly. Half the trouble with overweight people is that they eat so fast they hardly taste what they eat, and they end by eating more than they really want. Make dinner time a leisure time. Give the last bite time to hit bottom before you take on another one. Tell the kids funny stories instead of yelling at them. Try to recall the last nice thing your wife said to you. Grandma was right about another thing, too, when she told you to sit up and not slump at the table. An erect posture while eating also helps you cut down the quantity of your meal.

10. *The toughest on*e — obey the first nine rules.

Don't Count Calories — Count The Pounds

A bio-chemist could devote 16 hours a day to studying your eating habits and come up with an accurate count of your calorie intake.

Fortunately, we do not need a bio-chemist to add and subtract our calories. The problem is simple. It has only been made complex by authorities who want to impress you with their immense stores of knowledge of the subject. If you are overweight, you are taking on too many calories, more calories than your body is using in its normal daily activities. To keep from prescribing a starvation change in your calorie intake, I have already outlined a program of exercises to increase the calories you burn away.

The objective now is to find a new list of menus for you which will be satisfying, filling and realistic—the kind of change with which you will be able to live for the rest of your life. And of course the main idea is not to cut down on the *amount* of food you eat but the *kind* of food you eat.

Today's experiment is tomorrow's habit. Your taste buds may undergo a traumatic experience, if they haven't already been bombed out of existence by every extravagance on the grocer's shelf. But within two months, or less, a new world of delight will be opened to them. Non-fattening, healthful food is actually the main ingredient of the greatest epicurean discoveries.

You will be eating *better* and gaining *less*.

Most people are well aware of the pound-packing foods, or they think they are. A few have some idea of the foods preferred by nutritionists, or think they do. Later on in this chapter we will examine a list of the pound-packers and another list of the preferred foods, and your job will be simple—omit the pound-packers from your menus, substitute the preferred foods in their place.

But first let's strike a blow at, if you'll pardon the expression, the guts of the matter: *Meat* and *potatoes, bread* and *sweets.* Those are the four items on the average American dinner table which are 90 per cent responsible for most people being overweight. It would be unreasonable folly to suggest omitting them entirely, or even to cut down the quantity in any radical way. But there are several ways to keep them on the menu without wrecking a program of weight control.

Just follow these admonitions:

MEAT: The main culprit is beefsteak. There are more than 2,000 calories in a pound of prime rib. If you must have an occasional steak, trim away all the fat you can see. You will still be eating a ton which you can't see, but at least you're ahead of the game.

The least fattening cut of beef is beef round, so try to confine yourself to it.

But the best thing to do about beefsteak is to sub something else for it. Limit yourself to three entrees of meat a week, if you can, dining instead on fish or fowl. Veal loin, veal rib, leg of lamb, beef liver, dried beef in a careful casserole are other tasty ways out of the beefsteak problem.

Pork—including those juicy slices of breakfast bacon and the salt pork seasoning of vegetable dishes—is verboten, if you want to get anywhere with a weight-losing campaign. Instead, you may eat 2 slices Canadian smoked bacon with your morning eggs several times a week. It has 70 per cent fewer calories, and I think it's equally as tasty.

Gravy is out. Your might as well drink fat through a straw.

Summing up: Only lean beefsteak, and that rarely. Fish and fowl plenty. Canadian bacon OK. No gravy.

POTATOES: It's not so much the poor potato that adds on the pounds as what the cook does with it. A medium size spud, 2-3 inches thick, represents only 85 calories, and a whale of a lot of goodness—until the skin is trimmed away. Sliced and fried in lard or bacon grease it is damned near a lethal instrument. The one and only way to take your potato is baked, with a patty or two of corn oil margarine to make it palatable, skin and all. A once-every-two-weeks helping of French fries, using corn oil, is permissible.

Summing up: Baked potatoes only.

BREAD: The American variety is the world's most overrated food, a triumph of the ad man and the supermarket over your suffering stomach. The spongy, smooth-textured, comparatively tasteless product got that way because it is more easily merchandised when it "stays fresh longer." What it does is stay spongy longer. There's precious little in it in the first place to keep fresh, and in fact this streamlined Staff of Life contains no ingredients which you can't get in purer and better form in your regular meals.

Rye and whole wheat breads are superior to white bread in vitamin and protein content, but again not to such an extent that they are vital to a balanced menu.

Habit, however, is a powerful force. You may feel that if you can't have your bread and eat it too, then to hell with the whole thing. Gluten bread is your answer.

Gluten is the nitrogenous part of the flour of wheat which remains behind when the starch is removed by kneading the flour in a current of water. The end result is more expensive commercially, but so much lower in calories that it is the ideal substitute for people who are trying to lose weight.

Summing up: By omitting the store-bought variety, you are not missing much. Sub gluten bread and grow slender.

SWEETS: For the fellow who has a "sweet tooth," the farewell to candies, cokes and cakes is a tremendous sacrifice. However, the future is bright. The affliction is not congenital. A few months weaning and he can be cured for life. Meanwhile his hankering must be assuaged to some extent or we'll lose him entirely, something like the withdrawal of a dope addict. Part of the answer is honey, the best of all sweeteners. The rest of it is to concoct desserts which won't hit bottom like a bomb and turn into instant fat. We can also supply him with a substitute for milk shakes. (See the recipes in this and the succeeding chapter.)

Summing up: For day-to-day sweetener, and particularly for coffee and tea, use honey. Discover new desserts.

Now, that wasn't so bad, was it? You still have your meat and potatoes, bread and sweets, but you have them in sensible perspective. The sacrifices have been cut down to human proportions, as they should be if we hope to stick with a weight-control program. The entire range of your changed eating habits will follow this pattern. Now, let's take a complete reading first of all the foods you *can* eat before considering which foods you must forego.

BREAKFAST FOODS

eggs, boiled or poached

smoked Canadian bacon (occasionally)

eggs, soft scrambled in corn oil (occasionally)

melba toast

grapefruit—fresh fruit (see below)

cantaloupe and honey dew melon

calf kidney

coffee (sweetened by honey only)

Cream of Wheat (farina)

oatmeal

bran flakes (unsweetened)

corn grits (*not* hominy)

fresh orange juice

fresh strawberries, peaches, figs

canned tomato juice

FRUITS

apples

apricots

grapefruit

watermelon

canned pears, peaches (unsweetened)

applesauce (unsweetened)

lemons, oranges, tangerines

cantaloupe, honeydew melon

fresh strawberries, peaches, pears

pineapple (fresh and canned) and pineapple juice

VEGETABLES

artichoke (with olive oil and lemon juice)

asparagus

broccoli

cabbage

celery

eggplant

lettuce

squash

spinach

beets

onions (boiled)

endive

bean sprouts

string beans

brussel sprouts

cauliflower

cucumbers

green peppers

okra

tomatoes

radishes

carrots

turnips

baked potato

MEAT

beef round

smoked Canadian bacon

beef, calf or lamb kidney

calf brain

pickled pigs feet

rabbit

leg of lamb

veal loin, rib

calf liver

calf tongue

venison

dried beef

FISH

bass

bonito

finnan haddie

lobster

shrimp

bluefish

crabmeat

halibut

oysters (raw)

trout

FOWL

chicken

quail

pheasant

squab

DAIRY PRODUCTS

cottage cheese   skim milk

yogurt   buttermilk

(corn oil margarine, sparingly)   sherbet

BREAD

gluten bread   that's all, brother

I don't want to lecture you about the starving Armenians, but the above lineup of foods you *can* eat while losing weight would not win you any sympathy from the really hungry people of the world. Which, of course, is the whole point. If you go around hungry in an attempt to lose weight, the campaign will certainly not last long enough to do you any *permanent* good.

Now let's examine the other side of the coin:

THE POUND PACKERS

Breakfast Foods:

fried eggs   bacon, sausage, ham

corn flakes   shredded wheat

hominy grits

Dairy Products:

butter   cream

ice cream   homogenized milk

                                     cheeses (except cottage)

Fruits:

bananas   dried apricots

cranberry sauce   grapes

frozen strawberries   dry prunes, raisins

plums   fresh prunes

dried dates, figs

Fish:

herring   fried oysters

mackerel   dried squid

sardines

Vegetables:

green peas
kidney beans
sweet potatoes
lima beans
corn

fried, boiled potatoes
navy beans
hominy
succotash

Meat and Fowl:

beefsteak (most cuts)
goose
pork

turkey
duck

Miscellaneous:

bakery products
salad dressing
  (except olive oil-vinegar)
syrup
pickles
spaghetti, macaroni
candies, jellies

catsup
cocoa

nuts (except walnut)
marmalade
popcorn
alcoholic beverages*

*Note: Two martinis are caloric equivalent of one-pound sirloin steak

* * * *

There are 52 items listed in the Pound Packer section. Granted that they represent a huge hunk of living, there still remains 80 items of preferred foods which you may substitute.

Common sense is the only other guide you need. If you are 30 or more pounds overweight, you will have to cut down drastically on the *amount* of food you eat for the first few weeks as well as changing the kind of food you eat. On the other hand, if you are only 10-15 pounds overweight and you are following one of the exercise programs I have prescribed, you may only need to cut the Pound Packers from your menus.

Thousands of excellent dishes may be prepared from the list of preferred foods with the guidance of an ordinary household cook book. The list of recipes I suggest below have two advantages: 1) They are all tasty, and 2) most of them can be handled by the guy who doesn't know a cheese grater from an egg beater.

TUNA FISH MEXICAN STYLE

1 can tuna fish

½ avocado

1 tablespoon chopped onion

½ chopped jalapeno pepper

1 chopped tomato

3 onion rings, 3 radishes

2 small romaine leaves

1 teaspoon chopped parsley

Mix the chopped tomato, onion, jalapeno and parsley together and place on dinner plate. Chop the avocado over the mixture, top with tuna hunks and garnish with onion rings, romaine leaves and radishes.

SALMON STUFFED AVOCADO

1 cup (8 ounces) canned pink salmon

1 avocado

1 tablespoon finely chopped onion

1 tablespoon chopped parsley

2 tablespoons chopped tomato

1 tablespoon mayonnaise

2 slices jalapeno pepper

2 tablespoons lemon juice

¼ head lettuce

salt and pepper

Cut the avocado in half lengthwise, remove the seed and peel. Sprinkle with lemon juice. Combine the salmon, onion, parsley and tomato and toss with mayonnaise, salt and pepper. Pack mixture in seed cavity of avocado halves and garnish with one slice of jalapeno each.

SHRIMP COCKTAIL

8 shrimp

1 tomato

¼ lemon

1 cup catsup

2 tablespoons horseradish

Mix catsup and horseradish to taste and place in small bowl in center of dinner plate. Surround bowl with cold shrimp garnished with tomato wedges and lemon slices.

POACHED EGGS CREOLE

5 tomatoes	2 eggs
7 jalapeno peppers	4 tablespoons corn oil margarine
cream cheese (pkg.)	1 cup water, salt and pepper

Mix (preferably in blender) 4 tomatoes, 6 peppers and margarine with one cup of water, adding salt and pepper to taste. Cook mixture over low flame 15-20 minutes. Poach eggs as desired, put on plate and pour creole sauce over. Garnish with wedges of cream cheese and tomato and pepper slices.

HIGH PROTEIN CHICKEN DINNER

chicken breast (1 per person)	2 carrots
1/2 cup chopped onion	1/2 cup chopped celery
1 tomato, lettuce leaves	3/4 tablespoon chicken base

Put chicken breast in water, salt and pepper and bring to boil, turn flame low and simmer for 15 minutes. Add carrots cut in large pieces, onion, celery and chicken base and simmer 20 minutes longer, until vegetables are done. Remove chicken and serve on plate with lettuce and tomato. Serve vegetable and liquid as soup.

BEEF ON A SHINGLE
(Famous In World War II)

1 1/2 tablespoon flour	1/2 package dried beef (8-ounce pkg.)
1/2 cup skim milk	1 tablespoon corn oil
2 slices gluten bread	

This is a quick one. Toast two pieces of bread first. Pour oil in skillet over medium range heat, add bits of dried beef and stir for 2-3 minutes. Sprinkle on flour and salt a little at a time to avoid lumping. Add skim milk and keep stirring until the whole mess is pretty thick. Pour over toast.

THE FAT MAN'S CAKE
(Soya Muffins)

1½ cup soya flour

1½ teaspoon vegetable salt

3 tablespoons brown sugar

¼ cup floured raisins

2 teaspoons baking powder

2 fresh eggs

1 tablespoon grated orange rind

1 tablespoon corn oil

¼ cup floured walnuts

Sift flour, baking powder and salt. Separate eggs, beat yolks until very light and frothy. Add sugar, orange rind, milk and oil to yolks and mix well. Pour egg mixture into dry ingredients and mix. Add raisins and nutmeats and mix thoroughly. Fold in egg whites beaten stiff. Pour into small muffin tins and bake in slow oven (300 degrees) for 35 minutes.

DELMONTEQUE DELIGHT

1 slice watermelon (use only seedless portion)

1 slice papaya (or 1 pineapple ring)

1 strawberry
juice of 2 oranges

1 slice cantaloupe

1 slice honeydew melon

3 tablespoons cottage cheese
honey

In a fruit bowl, chop the fruit and stir in the orange juice, top with cottage cheese and the strawberry. Add as much honey as desired.

WHEAT GERM CAKE MUFFINS

1 cup wheat germ

1 egg

1 cup whole wheat flour (sifted)

¼ cup honey

¼ cup chopped pecans (optional)

⅔ cup skim milk

¼ cup soy oil

2½ teaspoons baking powder

½ cup raisins

Sift whole wheat flour and baking powder with pinch of salt, add other ingredients, mix, and bake in muffin tin for 25 minutes with oven at 400 degrees. Serve with scoop of sherbet.

Step Up To The Health Bar

It's only logical that the march of science, keeping one stride ahead of the race for the fast buck, should produce new discoveries in weight control. The pressures for physical excellence in the booming world of sports and the commercial jackpot awaiting the product which rescues the fat housewife are equally responsible.

On the commercial front, an all-purpose 900 calorie liquid substitute for food has been followed by 99 other mixtures, of which none are harmful and a few worthwhile.

The astronauts eat their suppers in flight out of a toothpaste tube, and there has been a suggestion that the next capsule for the moon be made of edible stuff. George Orwell and 1984, here we come.

Somewhere in this profusion of excesses and extremes, help is available for the average guy who wants to get back to his normal weight *and stay there*. Not even the sponsors of Metrecal advertising suggest that you may want to stick with their product forever. Benzedrine aside, athletic coaches are helpful to us because of their pragmatism —does it work, or doesn't it? From their ranks has come an unqualified "yes" on great natural boosters such as honey, wheat germ and a protein food supplement.

This plunges us into the subject of "food faddism," a phrase which dieticians utter with a shudder. Their target is the nut who stuffs himself to the gills with every new gimmick on the health food market, the fellow who ignores the fundamentals of good eating and thinks he has found a magic potion. But he is no more at fault than the qualified food experts who issue a blanket condemnation of food supplements, in whatever amounts. Both extremes are wrong.

Let's state the case for honey, wheat germ and protein powder simply, so that there can be no contradiction from any quarter.

1. Honey is a pleasant way to consume carbohydrates as an energy source, and it has a 30 per cent lower calorie count than sugar. There is a dispute about the ease with which the body dissipates the carbohydrates from honey, with much evidence indicating they are *not* converted into body fat.

2. Wheat germ (and wheat germ oil) is a proven source of energy which increases efficiency in physical activity.

3. Protein is not necessary for the *performance* of athletic exercise, but it is necessary for the growth of muscles, particularly in the non-athlete who begins a program of exercise.

Of those three statements, only the second will still be open to argument, and I think the experiments and conclusions of Dr. Thomas K. Cureton, director of the University of Illinois' Physical Fitness Research Laboratory, should clinch the case. Dr. Cureton put 16 middle-aged men on an exercise program, and eight of them were fed wheat germ oil in capsule form immediately after each workout. The other eight were given placebos, that is, capsules of vitamin-free substance. To rule out the psychological factor, none of the men was told what any of the capsules contained. At the end of eight weeks the men who had been taking wheat germ scored 50 per cent better on the exercise program than their germless compadres.

Dr. Cureton also experimented with a 40-year old university scientist over a period of seven years, charting his physical progress during extended exercise programs with and without wheat germ oil, and also during long instances of complete inactivity. The man scored progressively better when exercising, and when exercising with the benefits of the wheat germ supplement.

From all of these studies, I have concluded that the man who starts a program of exercise and improved eating habits can get a terrific boost from mixing a few drinks for himself. These can occasionally be substituted for an entire meal, particularly at breakfast and supper time. "Bulk" is such a distasteful word I hesitate to mention it, but these drinks are so flavorful that their filling quality might go unnoticed. The ingredients are available nowadays at most supermarkets.

I don't recommend one brand over another, but I do suggest that you equip yourself with a high-speed blender ($20 up) for the better enjoyment of these recipes.

MAINSTAY SPECIAL

10 strawberries (or sliced fresh peach, pear, pineapple as you wish)

1 tablespoon high protein powder

6 ounces skim milk

2 raw eggs

½ cup crushed ice

2 heaping tablespoons honey

1 teaspoon wheat germ

Place all the ingredients in a blender for two minutes, serve in 16-ounce glass. (Cocktail shaker may be used, a pretty good workout in itself.)

VITAMIN C COOLER

(A good sub for breakfast)

6 ounces grapefruit or orange juice

1 tablespoon of honey

1 teaspoon wheat germ

1 tablespoon protein powder

5 drops lemon juice

½ cup crushed ice

Place ingredients in a blender for two minutes, serve in a 12-ounce glass.

QUICK ENERGIZER

6 ounces orange juice

½ banana (slightly overripe)

1 tablespoon wheat germ

¼ cup crushed ice

1 tablespoon honey

Place ingredients in a blender for two minutes, serve in a 10-ounce glass.

TUTTI FRUITTI SHAKE

4 ounces orange juice

2 tablespoons honey

¾ cup crushed ice

assorted chopped fruit (banana, strawberry, apple, cantaloupe, watermelon, orange, pear, peach)

Place in a blender for two minutes, serve in 10-ounce glass.

POPEYE PUNCH

4 ounces orange juice

1 cup parsley

1 cup crushed ice

1 cup spinach

juice of ½ lemon

Place in blender for two minutes, serve in 10-ounce glass.

VITAMIN A SPECIAL

6 ounces carrot juice

1 tablespoon honey

½ cup crushed ice

juice of ½ lemon

1 tablespoon protein powder

Place in blender for two minutes, serve in 10-ounce glass.

THE VEGETARIAN

(requires automatic juicer)

½ cucumber

1 cup parsley

½ beet

5 carrots

1 cup spinach

2 celery stalks

Put ingredients through juicer, stir 30 seconds in blender, serve in 10-ounce glass.

YEAST ON THE ROCKS

(An antidote for hangovers)

3 tablespoons brewer's yeast

1 tablespoon honey

6 ounces skim milk

½ slightly overripe banana

Place in blender for two minutes, serve in 10-ounce glass.

How Sophia And Marlene
Got That Way—Salads

I have often been plagued by females with questions about "the secret foods of the stars." The ladies are convinced that surely Hollywood has its own methods for preserving gals whose figures are their fortunes. Well, there are no secret foods, and though the movie makers have developed highly scientific programs for weight loss they are simply variations of pushing yourself away from the dinner table.

There is, however, one trick we can pick up from the Hollywood beauties. It is a ruse which also happens to be a requirement of the gourmet—the salad dish.

Sophia Loren, and other Italian beauties who are inclined to fulsomeness and ravioli, have found a way to have their spaghett and their curves, too. The trick is to begin with a huge salad as the first course of the meal. In addition to being an aid to digestion, the low-calorie salad leaves less room in the appetite for the fattening courses which follow.

I once had the pleasure of dining with the most glamorous of women, Marlene Dietrich, at Cannes. Miss Dietrich began with a lettuce and tomato salad heaped high enough to hide a rose bush. She seasoned it with lemon juice and olive oil. Her main course of rare prime rib was moderate in size, followed by a dessert of sliced apples and honey, and a few pieces of ricotta cheese.

In gourmet fashion, a salad should be served as a separate and introductory course. Of course the French idea is to use the salad as an enticement for the greater pleasures to come, rather than an end in itself.

Most men regard the fresh greenery with disdain and call it "rabbit food." If they eat it at all, they dabble at it along with the rest of the meal. They are missing a good bet to lose weight the easy way.

The following recipes are merely introductory. There are hundreds of taste-quenching varieties.

SHRIMP SALAD

20 shrimp, cooked and cut to bite-size

1 cup diced celery

1 hard-boiled egg

1 sliced tomato

1 teaspoon lemon juice

1/2 cup mayonnaise (with teaspoon powdered pimento)

1/4 cup sliced olives

salt, pepper, celery salt

Mix shrimp, mayonnaise, lemon juice and celery. Garnish with sliced hard-boiled egg and olives, serve on tomato slices.

TUNA STUFFED TOMATOES

1 can tuna fish

2 tablespoons chopped onion

1 teaspoon chopped parsley

leaves of 1/4 head lettuce

2 tomatoes

1 tablespoon mayonnaise

1/2 jalapeno chopped pepper

salt and pepper

Cut tomatoes halfway in four sections and scoop out the insides. Mix tuna fish, onion, parsley, mayonnaise, jalapeno and place on lettuce bed. Garnish with slices of cantaloupe or honeydew melon.

POLYUNSATURATED MAYONNAISE

2 egg yolks

1/4 cup olive oil

1 tablespoon lemon juice

3/4 cup corn oil

1/4 teaspoon salt

Mix eggs and salt in automatic mixer and add oil slowly from a tablespoon until mixture starts to thicken. Add lemon juice after adding the oil.

Note: pink mayonnaise can be made with 1 tablespoon of powdered pimento, and "hot" mayonnaise with a New Orleans flavor can be made by adding 1 teaspoon of dry mustard and dashes of Louisiana hot sauce.

CRABMEAT SALAD

8 ounces (1 cup) crabmeat	1/4 cup chopped celery
1 chopped hard-boiled egg	1 tablespoon hot mayonnaise
1/4 head lettuce	1 tomato

Mix crabmeat, egg, celery and hot mayonnaise, serve on leafy lettuce, garnished with tomato quarters.

RAW VEGETABLE SALAD

1 cup finely chopped spinach	1 cup grated carrots
1 sliced tomato	1 hard-boiled egg
1 tablespoon raisins	1 cup grated beets
2 ounces olive oil	juice of 1 lemon

Place spinach, carrots, beets on separate parts of dinner plate, with tomato slices spaced between. Cut egg into four wedges and place in center. Put the raisins in the carrot portion. Sprinkle olive oil and lemon juice over the entire plate.

HARD-BOILED EGG SALAD

2 hard-boiled eggs	2 tomatoes
1/4 head lettuce	1 tablespoon parsley
4 onion rings	4 slices jalapeno pepper
1 tablespoon olive oil	juice of 1 lemon

Arrange alternate quarter wedges of tomato and egg on bed of lettuce. Garnish with onion rings, sprinkled parsley and jalapeno. Add oil and lemon dressing.

How To Relax At Home And Office

Among the problems of doing right by your physical self, the question of relaxation may be the biggest puzzler. Most men, upon arriving home with all nerve ends quivering, say the hell with it and proceed to get swacked on martinis or manhattans, which are fattening as well as befuddling.

Pity the poor folk of bygone centuries. The hewers of wood and the drawers of water never knew the blessings of air conditioning, the non-stop freeway, or one part vermouth to four parts gin. But neither did they suffer the malaise of today's cliff-dweller, the tense-as-tinfoil office worker. Nervous tension is as bad as the man on television says it is, and at one time or another most desk-bound people are plagued by it.

Taut emotions result in taut muscles. The solution is simple: relax your muscles to relax your nerves. You need to learn but four uncomplicated physical maneuvers to rid yourself of these tension troubles at the office.

But first let's consider the moment you arrive home at the end of a hard day. What I am about to propose will be received with hysterical protest, I'm sure, but nevertheless, here it is: Do a few pushups, situps, sidebends and half knee bends. Or at least go for a walk down a couple of blocks and back. Then spend 10 minutes in a bathtub of hot water, so hot that you have to ease into it. If your wife has some bath oils, use them. They are relaxing as well as fragrant, proving that you can get stinking without benefit of alcohol.

A hot shower will not do the job—you need the restfulness of a tub. Rinse off with warm water from the shower spray. Then, using the thickest towel in the house, rub down past the point of dryness to stimulate your circulation. Now, brother, you are *relaxed!* Try not to fall asleep before supper.

Quite a few paragraphs in this book have ridiculed sport as a physical conditioner. Now, on the subject of a businessman's relaxation, we have come to its rightful place. The secret here is to select a field of recreation you enjoy—golf, fishing, hunting, tennis, or whatever—*and assign yourself to it without guilt.* Such a pastime is not a luxury but a prescribed necessity if you wish to stay healthy and *perform more effectively at your work.* An exception to this rule is the man whose competitive fires burn so brightly that when he turns to sport he merely sets up another category of tension. Cherish the positive aspects of your game, ignore defeats. The poorest duffer touring 18 holes of golf can't fail to hit *one* good shot, and the memory of it should be carried home with him. You went fishing and caught no fish? Dwell on the pleasure you got from being in the fresh air and the raw elements. Simpler pastimes may suffice—put up a ping pong table in your backyard, or a horseshoe pit.

At the office, you should first consider the ideal non-exercise as a route to relaxation. This suggestion, particularly aimed at executives who spend up to 12 and 15 hours a day in concentration on business, is the mid-afternoon nap. About an hour after lunch, put your feet up on your desk and try to doze for 15 minutes. There is a mistaken notion that such an interlude will make you foggy. The contrary is true. You will be fresh, as well as relaxed. After one such period of goofing off in mid-day, Thomas Alva Edison invented the light bulb.

It would help, of course, if you had your own office, and a phone that would unplug. "I am in conference, Miss Blue."

The higher up the executive ladder you are, it seems, the more eccentricities you are allowed. Where extroversion is the key to business, such as on Madison Avenue or in sales departments, the lowest clerk has latitudes. Admen popularized the bongo board (a three-foot plank balanced on a rolling pin) and the Pica Poles (a variation of ski sticks) as acceptable office equipment. A later craze is the chinning bar near the top of a doorway. They are all fine, supposing that the man has the personality stature to indulge in them without self-consciousness (another source of tension).

What the average office worker needs, however, is a simple group of exercises he can perform right there at his desk—to keep tension and tiredness from striking him in the back of the neck like an ax.

The trouble spots are the trapezius muscles which extend across the back of the neck and shoulders, the lower stomach muscles, and the inside thigh muscles.

It's very easy to give them a slight going-over:

1. The Shrug And Stretch

In your desk chair, hold arms straight down toward floor. Raise shoulder blades as if trying to touch them to your ears, until your fingertips touch the edge of your chair seat. Hold for a count of five. Next, drop your shoulders as far as you can, point your chin at the ceiling and try to make your neck as long as a giraffe's. Hold for a count of five. The stretch should reward you with a few snap-crackle-pop sound effects from the region where de head bone connected to

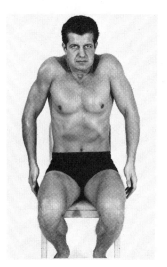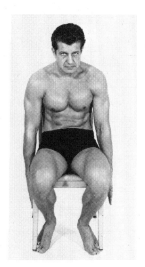

The Shrug And Stretch

de neck bone. Do three repetitions of the Shrug-Stretch three times a day, or whenever tension grabs you.

2. The Slump And Press

In your desk chair, hold arms straight but not rigid and rest your wrists on your knees as you lea.. forward. Let your head fall until your chin is on your chest, and arch your back like a cat's, tensing muscles for a count of five. Relax muscles and stay in that position for a count of two. Next grip the back edge of your chair seat, press shoulders back until shoulder blades seem to touch, and lift your chest. Hold for a count of five. Start over with the first part of the exercise and do three repetitions of this combination. Repeat at least three times a day. The important thing is to do them *before* tension sets in.

3. The Knee Up

Get a good grip on the front edge of your chair seat. Extend your legs straight, knees stiff, ankles together, and bring your knees up toward your chest slowly. Next, slowly straighten your legs again. Do not let your feet touch the floor, and try to keep your thighs from supporting the weight of your legs as much as you can. Without pausing, repeat the exercise. Do five repetitions at each session the first

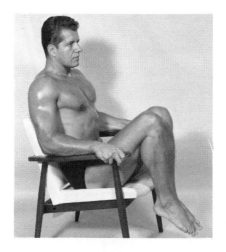

The Knee Up

day, increasing gradually until you can do 10 without effort. You should find time for at least four sessions a day.

This is a variation of the Knee Out (See page 19) and like its big daddy is aimed at reducing the paunch below the belt line. It also works the muscles on the inside of the thighs. As an office exercise, it is relatively worthless unless the knees are drawn up to straining point, adding a necessary third reaction, the compression of the upper stomach. Done properly it's a whale of a relaxer.

4. The Windmill Touch

Once again, your office environment will determine whether you can give this one a try in mid-day. A few brisk repetitions at home, before and after work, would be the next best thing, and still be effective.

Stand upright with feet slightly apart, arms outspread. Keeping arms rigidly opposite, bend left arm downward and alongside left leg. Your right arm should then be pointing at the ceiling. Bending your left knee and keeping the right leg reasonably straight, touch your left toe and return to starting position. Duplicate the exercise with right hand touching right toe. The movements should be done with deliberation, at a rate of one touch every three seconds. Begin with 10 to each side and increase by five daily to a goal of 25.

This exercise is directed at the muscles along the backs of the legs and at the oblique muscles in your sides. It also eases tension across the shoulders.

* * * *

Those are the keys to relaxation. If they all fail, my advice to you is to quit your job and get into another line of work.

I understand there's quite a good living to be had scrounging for shells in Tahiti.

A Crash Diet—The Egg And You

There are those amongst us whose impatience knows no bounds. They want results in a hurry. You can't tell such a man to relax and take a walk in the woods. He will say, "Bah! Humbug!"

You know the type:

"Miss Brown, get me Honk Kong."

"Yes, J.B."

When this fellow wants to lose weight he expects to tighten his belt two notches in two weeks. It so happens that I have just the thing for him—a 14-day crash program that will melt off 10-20 pounds, and perhaps leave him unable to stare an egg in the eye for months thereafter.

Barnyard fruit is the main ingredient of this diet, a batch of menus recommended (with important reservations) by one of the country's famed medical clinics. Before making further comments two points must be emphasized at the outset:

1) If you have the slightest history of major illness in your medical background, this egg onslaught should have the approval of your doctor. Even if you don't, a check with him would be wise. Perhaps there is a record of diabetes in your family. Remember—err on the side of caution.

2) The diet is for two weeks *only*. It does not follow that you can double your weight loss by doubling the length of the diet. The dim-

inishing returns make this idea foolish and in some cases dangerous.

On principle I am against short-term changes in.eating habits. In the long run they prove ineffective. There are, however, impressive psychological benefits in a crash program. The results are quickly measurable on your bathroom scale. A person who is considerably overweight may be so heartened by this initial success that he will continue to diet in a general way, back to normalcy.

Two to four exercise sessions within each week of the program will nearly double the effectiveness. Another point of importance is that you must not only abstain from anything not included in the diet but also eat what is assigned rather than doing without.

In a later chapter you will read that the latest studies of the cholesterol question warn against the continued high consumption of eggs, no matter how they are prepared. This is true. It's also another reason why the diet is only of two weeks duration. The evils of cholesterol must be fought over the years to have any bearing at all.

In this way the 14-day program may also be helpful. If you stick with it, I don't think you will mind cutting your egg intake in later months to three or four meals a week.

BREAKFAST: (Exactly the same for every day of the program.)
Half grapefruit, 1 or 2 eggs (if eggs are fried, use corn oil), black coffee.

MONDAY
LUNCH: Eggs, tomatoes, coffee.
DINNER: Eggs, combination salad, one piece of dry toast, half grapefruit.

TUESDAY
LUNCH: Eggs, half grapefruit, coffee.
DINNER: Steak, tomatoes, lettuce, celery, olives, cucumbers, coffee.

WEDNESDAY
LUNCH: Eggs, tomatoes, spinach.
DINNER: Two lamb chops, celery, cucumber, tomatoes, coffee or tea.

THURSDAY
LUNCH: Combination salad, half grapefruit, coffee.
DINNER: Eggs, cottage cheese, spinach, one piece of dry toast, coffee.

FRIDAY

LUNCH: Eggs, spinach, coffee.

DINNER: Fish, combination salad, one piece of dry
toast, coffee.

SATURDAY

LUNCH: Fruit salad. NOTHING ELSE.

DINNER: 14-ounce steak, celery, tomatoes, cucumbers,
tea or coffee.

SUNDAY

LUNCH: Cold chicken, tomatoes, half grapefruit.

DINNER: Chicken, tomatoes, cooked cabbage, carrots,
celery, vegetable soup, grapefruit, coffee or tea.

(NOTE: A certain amount of common sense must be used. For example, the vegetables without butter, the salad without oils, grapefruit without sugar or honey, no sweetener or cream in coffee or tea, and only the lean portions of steaks or chops. If you tire of wrestling halves of grapefruit, scoop the meat out with a knife and serve it on a lettuce leaf.)

Now You Can Be As Heavy As She Is — A Boost For The Thin Man

Does your girl outweigh you? Are the boys always putting you down in Indian wrestling? Do you look like a veteran of the Bataan Death March, and you don't have any medals?

The thin man's problem is really no kidding matter, though it invariably seems laughable to his portly brothers. Most slender fellows got that way due to a nervous indisposition. Until encroaching age changes his basic philosophy of life he is in no danger of becoming overweight. It therefore takes a concerted effort on his part to gain weight at all, but it can be done if he follows three principles, none less important than the others:

1) *Exercise.* This is a must to ward off the inroads of a Pear Shape physique.

2) *Accelerated Diet.* Though his fat friends may claim he stows food away like a horse, the thin guy just doesn't eat enough.

3) *Proper rest.* This, if you'll pardon the pun, is the sleeper. A weight-gaining program will be rendered practically useless unless Thin Man ups his nightly allotment of rest to nine hours. Ten would be better.

The greatest weight-gaining aid is milk, homogenized milk, not only because it is a pound packer but also because it's possible to drink so much of it during the day. A fellow who wants to gain should drink at least two quarts of milk a day, and it's not unreasonable to ask him to drink as many as three or even four quarts. He should get in the habit of downing a quart at one sitting, either with a meal or between meals.

Not all of the rules for gaining are the exact opposite of rules for losing weight. The thin man's penchant for candy bars and soft drinks between meals is equally ruinous to his cause. Whatever the effect of the added calories, it is more than dissipated by the lessening of appetite at mealtime.

Smoking is another detriment to his cause. If he cannot give up the habit entirely (as medical research advises), he can at least refrain from smoking for an hour before each meal. This alone will mean a tremendous increase in appetite.

Vitamin B tablets and brewer's yeast are other stimulants he needs to force him to pack away more groceries. One cold bottle of beer, and the emphasis here is on *one*, will also help just before dinner, particularly in the summertime.

Fresh fruit should be available for post-dinner snacks, especially ripe bananas and apples.

And most important of all add a *fourth meal* at night, one hour before bedtime. This can be a full-scale eggs-bacon-potatoes supper, a concentrated raid on the icebox, or a "meal" in terms of another quart of milk. For variety, and for real efficiency in nighttime weight-gaining, he can mix himself one of the following muscle-building drinks. These are standard mixtures at health clubs for the thin man.

MUSCLE PUNCH

8 ounces whole milk	1 ripe banana
2 tablespoons honey	1 teaspoon brewer's yeast
½ cup crushed ice	1 tablespoon protein powder

Mix ingredients, preferably in a blender, for two minutes, serve in a 12-ounce glass.

SUPPER BOOSTER

6 ounces whole milk

2 raw eggs

½ cup crushed ice

2 tablespoons honey

fruit in season (1 ripe banana, or ½ can pineapple chunks, or 10 strawberries, or 1 fresh peach)

1 teaspoon brewer's yeast

1 tablespoon high protein powder

Mix in blender for two minutes, serve in 16-ounce glass.

BREAKFAST BOOSTER

6 ounces orange juice

1 tablespoon honey

1 tablespoon protein powder

1 ripe banana

1 teaspoon brewer's yeast

½ cup crushed ice

Mix in blender for two minutes, serve in 10-ounce glass.

Cholesterol — A Bogeyman
To Be Feared

There has been remarkable progress in the treatment of heart disease, but most of the advancement has come in new surgery techniques—the salvage of a bad heart. Still in the laboratory stage is the ideal of a permanent mechanical heart.

Exercise is prescribed as both preventive and recuperative medicine for heart ailments, a fairly recent conception where most doctors are concerned.

But aside from this modern advance, medical scientists have precious little to tell us about this dread killer which claims 700,000 American men every year. In the last decade there has been only one breakthrough, in a study that had its beginnings 50 years ago.

It was a two-pronged discovery: 1) The incidence of a high cholesterol level among victims of atherosclerosis, and 2) The reduction of cholesterol levels by a change in diet.

Atherosclerosis is a $10 word for grandpa's hardening of the arteries.

Cholesterol is a body chemical produced by the liver for many varied uses. The one which concerns us is its role in transporting fats in the blood stream. You can't get along without it. Now research has disclosed that you'd better not have too much of it either. Cholesterol, as it moves through the blood stream, deposits itself just beneath the walls of the arteries, thereby narrowing the channel through which the blood flows. Cholesterol also tends to corrupt adjacent healthy cells, which develop scar tissue and further close up the artery. Normally, the excess cholesterol which could cause this trouble is disposed of naturally by the body. But when the cholesterol level is too high, it stays there and clogs up the works.

Scientists are now trying to prove a direct relation between this cholesterol clogging and high blood pressure, the way you increase the speed of water from a garden hose when you place your finger partway over the opening. Perhaps their research has been delayed because they can't walk up to a guy and say, "How about letting me use your heart for a garden hose, old buddy?"

Enough research has been completed, however, to point the way for the sensible man. In 1949 at Framingham, Mass, the United States Public Health Service undertook a large-scale controlled study of cholesterol related to heart attacks, beginning a 20-year chart on 5,-000 men and women between the ages of 30 and 59. The results should curl the hair on the back of your neck. From readings taken every two years, the study shows that a high level of cholesterol *quadruples* the risk of a heart attack, and the fatal chance is doubled if your cholesterol level is *only 20 per cent above normal.*

Under the auspices of New York City's board of nutrition, an Anti-Coronary Club was formed in 1957 and its 600 male members were put on a diet calculated to lower the cholesterol count. From 1958 through 1962, the 400 volunteers whose ages range from 40 to 59 had only four heart attacks. On the basis of the Framingham, Mass, figures, a total of 24 heart attacks could have been expected in the New York group. Did the diet change "save" 20 men? Research does not work that patly, but the evidence is there.

Dr. Ancel Keys of the University of Minnesota's school of public health is a world authority who has conducted international research in the study of cholesterol's relation to diet. In an experiment involving 12 men, Dr. Keys proved that a change in diet reduced their cholesterol levels by 20 to 47 per cent *within a month's time.* The higher the original reading, the greater the reductions.

Now, you ask, how do I know I have too much of this stuff?

Simple. Get your doctor to measure the cholesterol in your blood. The standard reading is in milligrams per 100 milliliters of serum. In America, the average cholesterol for men ranges between 180 milligrams (MG) per cent for a 20-year-old up to 260 MG at age 50. If your cholesterol level is above 250 MG, you are in a deadly bracket of the statistical column. If you're under age 30 and your reading is over 200 MG, the same is true.

Men from 20 to 70 should try to stay within a sliding scale of 170 MG to 200 MG.

Okay, you say, so I've got MG's coming out of my ears. How do I get rid of them?

The single most deadly cause of increased cholesterol, and the culprit which started the entire study in the beginning, is saturated fat. "Saturated" is a chemist's adjective to describe the connection of atoms. Saturated fat is a string of carbon atoms, each with two hydrogen atoms attached.

But if saturated fat is the bane, its cousin unsaturated fat is the boon. In unsaturated fat one of the atoms in the carbon string is minus one of its hydrogen hitchhikers, a circumstance which actually *lowers* the cholesterol level. Fats which have several carbon atoms minus the hydrogen hitchhikers are called polyunsaturated. Better yet.

The solution seems easy—lay off the saturated fats, load up on the unsaturated and polyunsaturated variety. As you might have guessed, this turns out to be one helluva job. The mainstays of America's famed "square meal" are loaded with saturated fats—beef, pork, butter, eggs; all dairy products except skim milk, buttermilk and cottage cheese; ordinary margarine, solid fats such as lard and hydrogenated shortening, plus the whole roster of flour products.

Sources of polyunsaturated fats are relatively few—fish, and other seafood, pecans, peanuts, walnuts, whole grains, liquid vegetable cooking oils, special margarines, and the natural oils from safflower, corn, cottonseed, sunflower and sesame.

Though there is no corollary between overweight and cholesterol (a thin man's cholesterol count may be too high, too), the list of do's and don'ts in diets for lowering cholesterol are almost identical to those for losing weight. Your best bet, then, is to re-read my chapter on weight control.

A reasonable request to ask of yourself is that you avoid excesses in the saturated fat foods. Trim away the visible fat from your meat. Substitue corn oil margarine for butter or the margarine you have been using. Fry your foods in liquid vegetable oil, if you fry them at all. Veal is relatively neutral in the saturated fat ratings. Olive oil has no effect one way or the other. Use fish as an entree several times a week.

You will note that I have singled out corn oil as my choice among the polyunsaturates. It is the most palatable of the bunch, far more so than safflower oil, which was once mainly used as a base for house-paint. There is no detectable taste difference between corn oil margarine and the old style margarines which have replaced butter on most housewives' shopping lists.

A special mention should be made of eggs, an important staple in any man's diet, and high in protein. It's possible that the consumption of two eggs daily will raise your cholesterol count by as much as 15 MG per cent. But this points up the mysterious way in which the body handles its cholesterol. It may be that you, in particular, have no cholesterol problem and therefore would not be troubled by egg intake. Check your doctor and find out where you stand on this cholesterol question.

The drug companies have been in a frenzy of research for a product which can lower the cholesterol count easily. So far the only things they have come up with are the polyunsaturated oils tricked up in an expensive package, and there are some doubts about the wisdom of forcefully inducing them into the body in this concentrated way. It is safer—and much cheaper—to add them to your cooking processes and everyday eating habits.

There are still many unresolved questions about cholesterol and its connection with atherosclerosis, and it becomes a problem of semantics and pure logic to present the so-far accepted truth of the matter.

For instance, some people with very high cholesterol levels never suffer from any vestige of the disease, and medical conservatives use this point to devaluate the importance of cholesterol as a factor. There is no logic to this refutation. There are also men who smoke two packs of cigarettes a day for 40 years and never develop lung cancer. To carry this argument further, perhaps you should have your son develop osteomelitis in his leg so he can grow up and hit a baseball like Mickey Mantle.

It should be enough warning to you when you consider the statistics alone: In any group of men, the half with the higher cholesterol counts will have three times as many deaths from heart attacks.

How To Fool Your Friends Into Thinking You Have Lost Weight— Conditioning From The Neck Up

Are you shocked when you stare into your shaving mirror every morning. Do you say to yourself: "Whatever happened to me? I'm not an old guy. Why is it I look like Walter Brennan's father?"

Your business suit conceals most of the wreckage, but what about the area from your shirt collar up?

Do rolls of fat spill over that collar, as if your worst enemy had knotted your tie? Or are you a turkey-wattle man, whose Adams apple fascinates the children when he drinks a glass of water. ("Daddy's got a yo-yo in his fwoat.")

Your appearance is only the half of it. How often have you been heard to complain that something, or somebody, gives you "a pain in the neck?" Your favorite expression may be less genteel in placing the pain considerably lower, but let's take one thing at a time. The significance of your "pain in the neck" should not be lost on you. Tension grabs us all. Even farm boys, whose anxieties were once limited to the weather, can now develop a fine case of the yips by considering crop allotments and price supports.

Exercise can't solve all of the civilized sources of tension, but it can certainly stop them from grabbing you by the neck. I believe that well-conditioned neck muscles will prevent most headaches and a great deal of fatigue.

Their effect on your appearance in positively dramatic. Firmness and good muscle tone in the neck will make you seem years younger than you are. This is a shortcut to physical conditioning which will amaze your friends.

As we shall see, there is no need to halt this trickery at the neck. There are 97 muscles in that fat face of yours, and we will get to them, too, but first the neck:

1. Necking In Bed

Lie crosswise on your bed, preferably alone, so that your head hangs backwards over the edge. Relax completely for a moment, then lift your head up and forward until your chin touches your breastbone, and return to original position, head lowered until you are staring at the wall behind you.

Start with eight repetitions and increase by one every session to a goal to a fast 50.

To remove rolls of fat, do the exercise as rapidly as you can. to build up a scrawny neck, do the exercise slowly in series of 10, resting 30 seconds in intervals.

You may find this routine expensive—after a month, none of your shirts will fit you anymore.

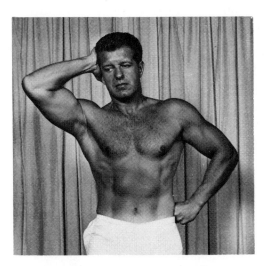

Necking With One Hand

2. Necking With One Hand

Place the palm of your right hand against your right temple. This is sometimes know as the "Oi vey!" position, or "Don't tell me that last check bounced." Put your left fist on your left hip. Resisting strenuously with your right hand, force your head sidewards toward right shoulder. You may have to bend slightly to the right at the waist to get there. Now, resisting with your neck muscles, push your head upright again. Repeat five times, then switch hands and repeat the exercise to the left five times. Increase by one per session until you are doing 10 to each side.

3. Face Lifting Without Surgery

In the depression years I went to New York to interview a Swedish face-lifter. The lady had hopes of becoming an American face-lifter also, and I did this story about her for one of Bernarr MacFadden's magazines. It was her thought that, some 20 years before surgery would be needed, a person could avoid the whole thing by practicing a set of facial exercises. Her theory seemed logical to me and I began following her suggestions. Down through the years I have taken a terrific ribbing from my friends, but now we are all past 40 and they say I'm the only one who doesn't look it. This prospect should repay you for the wisecracks you'll hear.

There are 97 muscles in your face, give or take a tic or two, and the trick is to give most of them a workout in a minimum of time. The three facial exercises I recommend here were part of a complete conditioning program I set up for the star of a TV western series, who shall be nameless. This guy is 6-5 and promised he'd slug me if I ever mentioned it.

THE JOWL RUB — Using hair tonic or preferably an oily lotion with a lanolin base—to ease the wear and tear on your beard—rub upwards with the heels of your hands from the jawbone to your eyes. Start with 15 repetitions the first session and increase by one to a goal of 50. This is the exercise you need if you wish to erase the telltale signs of dissipation, those bags *under* the bags under your eyes. You will soon look innocent enough to return to Sunday school.

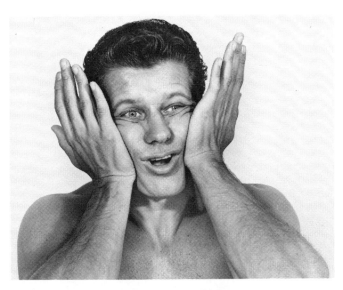

The Jowl Rub

THE BALLOON FACE — Puff your cheeks out as far as you can. Touch your tongue to the inside of your left cheek and then the right. Relax. Repeat 20 times the first session. Increase by one to a goal of 35.

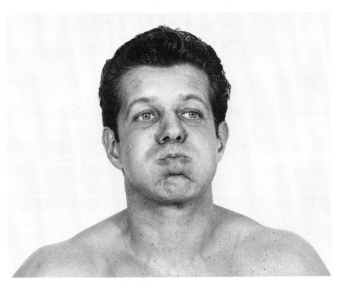

The Balloon Face

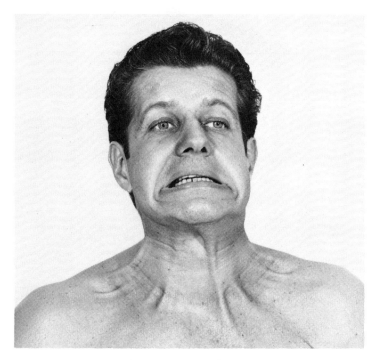

The Strong Yawn

THE STRONG YAWN—Thrust your chin down and outward and strain to keep it there for three seconds. Repeat 15 times the first session, and increase by one to a goal of 30.

4. The Mayonnaise Facial

Well, this may seem a bit much.

I doubt that I will recruit many followers in the following departure from the virile norm. Personally, I do not see that it is less manly to wish to look younger, or to take pride in glowing, clean, and healthy skin tones. You disagree. Step outside and say that.

The suggestion is a mixture of "mayonnaise" which you can apply to your face—like Al Jolson applied boot polish before he sang Mammy—and then wipe away, taking all of the dirt with it which your shower soap has missed, and leaving an undetectable residue of oil to relieve dryness of skin.

If it will make you feel more like Tarzan, whip the goop off with toilet paper instead of Kleenex.

The hard part is mixing the stuff in the first place. Here's how: In a mixing cup, place two fresh egg yolks and beat slowly. One tablespoon at a time, add ½ cup safflower oil, ½ cup sesame oil, and finally one tablespoon wheat germ oil. The ingredients should be slightly chilled before mixing. When the contents become thick and golden, add two drops of your favorite shaving lotion and 1 tablespoon of herb vinegar.

There's your mayonnaise. There is no better cleaning agent and no better treatment for dry skin. Mix up an extra batch for your girl friend or wife (or both) subbing perfume for the shaving lotion, and she will thank you for the best sunbathing lotion she's ever had.

As for you. Take it or leave it, but don't try it on tomatoes and lettuce. The stuff is practically inedible.

Hair Conditioning

There's no time for a man to recover his hair
that grows bald by nature . . .
Time himself is bald, and therefore to world's end
will have bald followers . . .
What he hath scanted men in hair, he hath
given them in wit . . .

William Shakespeare,
Comedy of Errors, Act II, Scene 2

The above is a little uptown talk from which you may conclude that the best time to stop your own comedy of errors is in Act I—like, right now.

Most cases of baldness are unavoidable, but no one knows how large a percentage of men allow themselves to go bald through sheer negligence and hair-thinning habits. My barber friends tell me this percentage is high, an opinion which I view with suspicion because I have been hustled by too many barbers pushing special hair tonics. Scientists, even bald scientists, have been too disinterested to gather reliable statistics on the subject.

Men who consult me professionally for physical conditioning programs are often surprised when I inform them there are ways to 1) discourage baldness, and 2) slow down the graying process. For the latter there is even a special physical exercise.

There are no panaceas, of course, for the man who is already bald. He, as the expression goes, has had it.

It's the fellow who is only on the way to skinheadedness who may still be saved—and by just a few simple tips which are no trouble to observe. As follows:

1. Throw away your comb. Buy a pair of military hairbrushes. And insist on hog bristles. Any other kind of bristles, including the new synthetics, can do more damage to your hair than almost anything else. If your hair is naturally unruly so that you must use ·a pocket comb several times during the day, buy an extra pair of hairbrushes and keep them at your office, or in the glove compartment of your car.

2. Try to find time, either morning or evening, for 100 brush strokes through your hair. How many bald women do you see? Dames are forever brushing their hair. If you object to the brush act, think about the jokes waiting for the guy with the shiny dome.

3. Shampoo your hair once a week, using a lanolin-base shampoo. Bath soap is worse than no shampoo at all.

4. Never let the shower spray hit your head directly. Baseball players supposedly go bald because they perspire beneath those wool caps. A contributing factor is the eight-foot high shower nozzles in most athletic plants.

5 Make sure that your hair dressing contains no alcohol. An American's trust in nationally-advertised products is one of the world's great misplaced faiths. Hair *oil* is your best bet, plus a dab of lanolin hairdressing.

Admittedly, any set of rules for preventing baldness is a heads I win, tails you lose proposition. If the expert's advice doesn't work, he can always tell the victim he would have gone bald no matter what he did. All I can tell you is that I've seen these stratagems work wonders for men who were beginning to get a little thin on top.

As for graying hair, I will pass on to you a hard-to-believe bit of advice I received 22 years ago from Bernarr MacFadden. He told me to stand on my head five minutes every day to keep from going gray. Eight years ago the silver threads among the gold started to show and I promptly went upside down. I'm on the long side of 40 now and I

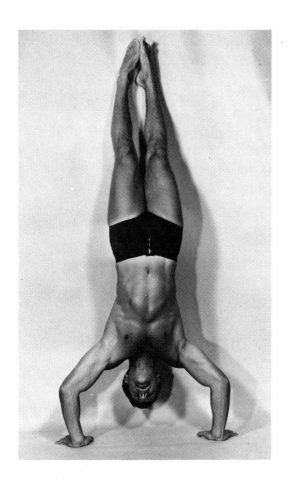

haven't gray hair one, unlike my father who was silver-thatched in his 30's.

The theory, of course, is that the upsetting aid to circulation will keep your locks their natural color. I don't know if there is any scientific basis in fact for the theory. All I know is that it works.

Place a pillow on the floor, a comfortable distance from the wall, and get those feet up there, heels to wall, even if you have to have help. Like other exercise, it requires moderation at the beginning—only a minute the first day, graduating to five.

Prehaps you'll decide this is too much trouble. As has been noted before, all cats are gray in the dark.

Exercise For The Heart Patient

Until recently a heart attack relegated the victim to the life of a
semi-invalid. If he was wealthy he installed an elevator in his home to
dodge the stairs; a ramp replaced the front steps. If he was poor he
retired from work, settled into a rocking chair on the front porch and
swatted flies—gently. Family relatives kicked in for the groceries.

In a way, it's a shame this fine old dodge is a thing of the past.
Doctors are now putting heart patients through a more strenuous life
than they had ever known before, beginning after a two or three
month period to allow for recovery from the initial damage. It is
amazing to me that the medical profession has not engaged itself in a
program of research to prove statistically the benefits of exercise for
both heart attack victims and for the general cross-section of males
who will be nearly decimated by coronary disease. Doctors of course
are doing wonderful jobs individually with their patients, following
the leads of the giants of their profession such as Dr. Paul Dudley
White of Boston, Dr. Joseph Wolffe of the Valley Forge Heart Hospital, Dr. Warren Guild of Harvard, and past American Medical
Association president Dr. Edward L. Bortz.

It remained for such lay groups as the Cleveland YMCA to under-
take a concerted program of careful exercise for heart patients and
to prove over a number of years its savings effect. The results at
Cleveland have been startling even to the proponents of physical activ-

ity.The program got its origin from the doctor who told municipal executive William Rogers that he should take exercise. Rogers had just recovered from the second of two heart attacks spaced twenty years apart. William Cumler, physical director of the Cleveland YMCA, put Rogers on a gradually increasing schedule of jogging, swimming and calisthenics. His first step was to walk across the swimming pool in chest-high water. At the end of the program, Rogers was jogging a mile, swimming a mile and doing a half hour of calisthenics *every day*. That was eight years ago. Rogers is now in his late 60s and has never felt better or more energetic in his life.

The success of this one man snowballed into a "Cardiac Club," which includes 30 graduates who previously had suffered heart attacks and over 200 businessmen who want to make sure they never have one. Dr. Herman Hellerstein, a research cardiologist at Western Reserve University, led a team of scientists into the Y to measure the results. Hellerstein found that Cardiac Clubbers were in better shape than the other Y members who were classified as normal.

The key to the idea is graduality. Some of Cumler's Club members had so little strength at the beginning that 10 seconds on a treadmill taxed their capacities. The next day they went 20 seconds. At the end they were running and swimming miles, for the first times in their lives.

Completely destroyed was the old notion of the heart as a fragile instrument. It is now recognized that the heart is mainly a muscle, and like any other muscle it can be conditioned and revitalized and ultimately toughened. Apparently "healthy" men, even as you, really have no guarantee that their hearts can withstand a crisis. An emotional shock, a sudden sickness, an automobile accident can make emergency demands which only a strong and conditioned heart can withstand.

Dr. Wolffe of Valley Forge says: "The heart gains strength through work. Regular exercise, with periods of rest, is the most important measure against disease of the heart and premature aging."

Dr. Bortz, former AMA chief, says: "It begins to appear that exercise is the master conditioner for the healthy and the major therapy for the ill."

Dr. White, the heart specialist who treated Eisenhower, says: "Even where the symptoms of coronary thrombosis still exist, some sort of exercise is generally advisable."

The only question remaining, then, is what *kind* of exercise is feasible for the heart patient? If you have already suffered a heart attack, you won't need my insistence that you consult your doctor before undertaking anything you have not been doing before. As it is you probably call him for advice before walking to the kitchen for a glass of water. You may need his assurance that you *can* begin a mild program of activity designed to regain your former strength and get in better condition than you have ever been before.

Here is a list of mild activities which can start you on the road back:

Deep Breathing: This is an important basic for any activity you decide to pursue. A series of 10 deep breaths several times a day will improve the tone of the diaphragm, which results in its better function as the piston of a pump, not only for bringing oxygen to the lungs with the removal of carbon dioxide, but also for the suction of blood into the heart.

Walking: (See page 35) This can develop into a vigorous enough exercise for anyone, as you increase pace and distance. It's an excellent time for your deep breathing requirements, too.

Hiking: A further acceleration of walking, because it entails getting into the countryside and negotiating uneven ground. As your powers increase, alternate stretches of jogging.

Cycling: Dr. White so favors this exercise that he and his wife ride bicycles through Ireland and France on their vacations. A bit of fun can be added if you buy a bicycle built for two (about $100). All neighborhood cycle shops now feature them. Should the traffic in your area make cycling dangerous, get a kid's used bike and anchor it to the floor in your garage. The main thing is to get your legs moving again.

Light Gardening: Notice I say "light" gardening. Some of the requirements of keeping a yard and garden beds in shape would fell a field hand. Start with a workout on a self-propelled lawn mower, and advance to weeding the garden and lawn. If your nervous system can withstand a battle with crab grass, your physique can, too.

Horeshoes and Shuffleboard: It's no accident that these are the favorite pastimes in Saint Petersburg, Florida, the famed retirement haven. A concrete shuffleboard court in your back yard is not an unreasonable expense; investigate it. Pitching horseshoes is also a highly competitive form of light exercise. The stakes should be 40 feet apart, with a 10-foot handicap for the ladies.

Swimming: You may have to start by merely walking through the water, but the main thing is to start. This is perhaps the best all-round conditioner possible for you. You should give some thought to installing a pool of your own in the backyard. In most parts of the country they now cost less than a new car. For best value and swimming room, pick an oval shape 17 feet wide and 32 feet long, with depth ranging from 8½ feet to 3 feet, nine inches. One of these costs about $3,200, and you might be able to get a discount by having it built in the off-season.

* * * *

From any of these beginnings you can advance to light calisthenics in your home, such as a half knee bend with both hands gripping the back of a straight chair. (See page 33.) From there, it is not far to a fullscale workout—situps, pushups and the works.

The goal can be achieved. You have the examples of hundreds of men before you. Just remember that the stakes are your life and your death.

The Lieberman Trot—Your Bedroom Running Track

In one of Xenophon's light-hearted reports on life in Athens, circa 400 B.C., Socrates was asked for the secret of his vitality. How was it that he stayed fresh in spirit and keen of wit, on into the conversational hours of the night?

"Because," said Socrates, "I dance every morning."

"It's true," a friend said. "I found him doing it and I thought he'd gone mad. But he talked to me and I tell you he convinced me. When I went home—I did not dance; I don't know how; but I waved my arms about."

Socrates lived to age 70 and for all we know might be going yet, if he hadn't downed that cup of hemlock, so anything the old boy did to insure longevity is worth noting.

A friend of mine in Houston, Attorney Seymour Lieberman, insists he knows the Socratic answer, which has lain dormant lo these 2,400 years. The President's Council of Youth Fitness thinks he does, too. After he wrote to them about his exercise, the committee included it as a vital part of its Adult Program. Lieberman now is one of the directors of a $200,000 study of his idea.

Lieberman's solution arose when he tried to work out a plan to get himself back in shape. He knew that doctors were unanimous in their approval of exercise as a deterrent to heart disease and other ills. But if they suggested any specific exercises at all, Lieberman noted that few of them were practical for the average, hurried businessman.

His own background had a great deal to do, I suspect, with the answer he found. Certainly it did in his adherence to it. Lieberman was a Big Ten track star in his college days at the University of Illinois and Loyola of Chicago, where he got his law degree. In later years he remained close to sports by serving as president of the South Texas AAU, then helped form the new United States Track and Field Federation. But, at 35, like quite a few of his contemporaries, Lieberman had gone to pot. Then began his investigation, spurred by a succession of heart failures among his clients and business associates.

Liebermam discarded golf as too time-consuming, swimming ditto as well as expensive (though he now has his own pool), and flirted idly with the notion to start a program of calisthenics. He vetoed the calisthenics because his problem was not one of overweight or physique—he wanted to condition his heart and his entire arterial system as well as his lungs, not trim pounds or build flattering muscles.

His basic answer then, the only thing that was left, was running. Every medical man recommended running. The problem was *where* and *when*. The idea of running through a public park in a sweat suit or track underwear did not appeal to him. "People would think I was some kind of nut," Lieberman says. No, leave that morning roadwork to the prizefighters . . .

Suddenly it came to him. His mind's eye saw a boxer, dancing lightly on his toes in the gym, punching at shadows. Lieberman, who like all lawyers has a talent for complicating things, put his discovery into an equation: Time = Distance.

Trackman Lieberman knew that it takes approximately eight minutes to jog a mile. *"Why,"* he asked himself, *"can't a guy jog in his own bedroom, or up and down the hall, for eight minutes, and cover a mile just the same?"*

Thus was born the Lieberman Trot, what its modest inventor believes to be the perfect exercise, bringing into play 300 separate movements of the body. And it is also akin to the exercise a doctor requires in a physical examination to check the efficiency of the heart by measuring the time it takes to return to normal after jogging a few times.

The only equipment needed is a pair of soft sole (preferably rubber sole) slippers. I'll let Lieberman tell you the rest:

"Start the exercise by running slowly, no faster than a walk. You are merely attempting to run in slow motion, to move leisurely. And this is the pace you will keep throughout. The ball of the foot hits the floor first and then the heel comes down. Hold your chest high, your abdomen in. Keep the rest of your body as limp as a rag doll. Your arms and fingers should shake along with the flesh and muscles of your body.

"Move to and from a certain point in the room or hall. Every fourth or fifth stride, roll your head to the left and to the right as close to your shoulders as you can.

"By holding your abdominal muscles taut during the entire five minutes of the exercise, you will strengthen them, thereby enabling you to hold your abdomen in at all times with little effort.

"After two minutes of jogging, your heartbeat will increase. A normal pulse of 70 may go to 120 or more after five minutes. This is good. It is the rapidity of the flow of blood that takes care of your heart. The rapid beating develops the heart muscles. In this manner the heart becomes accustomed to rigorous demands and as a result will withstand sudden shock or the emotional strain that causes heart attacks.

"The rapid beating of the heart will bring about good blood circulation throughout the body. The smallest vein, and all the capillaries and their tiny muscles will go into action. The muscles in these veins and capillaries will develop and the blood will bring new life to the tissues in the extremities of your body. This means an actual retarding of the ageing process.

"Jogging causes the hipbone to move against the flesh and fat around it, creating a massage sufficient to remove excess weight from the hips. For example, the two types of athletes who have the smallest hips are track athletes and boxers, who train by running every day."

Lieberman's routine is not for the man past 50 who already has a diseased heart—unless that man has completed a milder program of conditioning and has his doctor's approval for the strain of jogging.

Begin by limiting your self to one minute—preferably, morning *and* night to get the results of the idea—the first day or two. Spend the rest of the week increasing gradually to two minutes at a stretch. The second week go from two to four minutes, the third week four to six, and the fourth week all the way to your indoor eight-minute mile.

If you practice the game of One-Upsmanship at the office, this jogging bit will give you dandy ammunition: "Oh, yes. I run a mile every morning and a mile at night."

As in other cases of increased physical capacity, jogging is its own reward—one minute today will lead you quite naturally to eight minutes at a stretch within a month. And no one can furnish you with clearer motivation than did Dr. W. W. Bauer, chief of the American Medical Association's Department of Health Education, when he said: "If any man wants to improve his physical condition, add to his health, increase his endurance and chances of living a longer, more satisfactory life, he should add running to his exercise regimen."

Socrates may have put it better, but he certainly would have agreed.

Put Muscle In Your
Golf Game

Among devotees, golf is not a way of life to be taken lightly. For instance, there is the case of the man whose partner, a 200-pounder, collapsed of a stroke on the 13th hole. He hoisted the stricken one on his shoulders, and when he reached the clubhouse bystanders were amazed.

"How'd you manage to carry him that distance?" the pro asked.

"Oh, it wasn't bad carrying him," the man said. "What wore me out was picking him up and laying him down between shots."

This is a fairly accurate illustration of the importance some men place on a round of golf, and it is no wonder that par-busting equipment and inventions make up a multi-million dollar industry. Though no golfer myself, I know enough about the game to suggest that the quickest and most startling way a golfer can lower his score is something that won't cost him a cent. It is, of course, exercise.

If you take a few tips from me—and from Jackie Burke Jr., Jimmy Demaret and Gary Player—you'll soon agree.

In the game of gentlemen's golf, grace was once the basic word. Bobby Jones' instruction book of the early 30's asked the beginner to think of the clubhead as a rock on the end of a piece of string describing a centrifugal arc. The modern touring pros have changed all that. The old groove is still the same, but there's a lot going on when the clubhead starts down. You hear-about "late-breaking wrists" and the "power zone," and the shots that call for punching the ball.

"The once-a-week golfer," says Jackie Burke, ex-champion of the Masters and the PGA, "has a built-in handicap. He is simply not in shape to play top golf. The average player poops out on the 15th hole or sooner. Unless he plays three or more times a week, the game itself won't get him in condition. But even daily golfers can improve their scores by a special set of exercise."

The five muscle areas which need help are in the hands, wrists, forearms, shoulder and thighs. By shoulders I mean the muscle across the top of the back and to the rear of the armpit. Stronger hands will solve many of the problems of achieving a firm but relaxed grip. Powerful wrists will allow you to start moving the clubhead later in the downswing, which is also where forearms muscles come into play.

Jack Nicklaus played in a foursome with Jim Brown, the All-NFL fullback of the Cleveland Browns, and afterward remarked: "If Jimmy could get his hands into the shot he'd drive the ball further than any man alive," This is the Nicklaus who astounded Britons with a 370-yard drive in the 1963 British Open.

The thighs are of prime importance to the middle-aged golfer. That's where your legs quiver when you stand over a putt on 18. The great Ben Hogan, his fellow pros believe, would still be winning championships if his legs, and his putting game, had not faltered.

Let's see how three great professionals handle these conditioning problems:

1. Jackie Burke Jr.

This son of a famous golfing father has developed the most efficient swing in the sport and is always striving for more distance— what he terms "natural distance"—provided by strength. In addition to daily situps to keep his waist supple, Burke concentrates on strengthening his hands and building the sloping muscles at the back of the armpits.

For his hands, Jackie carries a simple spring-grip set which costs about $1 in most sporting goods stores. He hangs it on the direction-

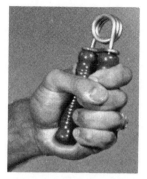

turn-signal handle in his car. Several times a day he does a series of 50 presses with each hand. (Someone starting this exercise could begin with 20 and gradually increase to 50.) Every couple of months, Jackie buys a new and stronger set. On occasion he has used a child's sponge-rubber ball, $2\frac{1}{2}$ to 3 inches in diameter, instead of the spring-grip.

To build the latissimus muscles for a strong follow-through, Jackie uses a towel-pull exercise, holding one end of the towel with both hands at waist level, feet slightly apart for balance. A partner holds firm to the other end of the towel and Jackie pulls it toward his waist with slow, steady strength. (See the V-Builder, Page 27.) He does 15 to 25 of these at each session.

A man careful of his health in all respects, Jackie eats a lot of lean steak, and includes fresh fruit in his diet daily. He carries an energy drink in a vacuum bottle in his golf bag—$1\frac{1}{2}$ tablespoons high protein powder, 6 ounces of fresh orange juice, 1 cup crushed ice and 2 tablespoons of honey mixed in a blender. He believes all golfers could benefit from this drink on the course when they start to feel tired.

There's one other recommendation from Jackie: Walk, do not ride, around the golf course. "The only exercise some golfers get," he says, "is holding onto the handlebars of a golf cart to keep from falling off."

2. Jimmy Demaret

This three-time Masters champion, and more recently a fine TV commentator of golf shows, is past 50 and yet still able to finish in

126

the top ten of any tournament. He has probably shaped the game of golf through strength more than any other pro.

Demaret's forte has always been powerful wrists and forearms, which he came by occupationally. As a youngster working in a golf shop, Demaret would buff 200 sets of clubs a day. Holding the clubs firm against the buffing machine brought into play the muscles which enabled him to "punch" the golf ball to a fortune in winnings and international fame.

As a kid, Demaret used a full swing, but he shortened it after he saw Walter Cruickshank and Walter Hagen. "A short backswing," he says, "gives you fewer movements and more consistency. It may cost you distance, but it gains you accuracy." Most of today's pros agree with him.

But a shorter swing demands a set of Demaret wrists and arms. Jimmy no longer has to man a buffing machine at his plush Champions Golf Club outside Houston, but he has a special exercise he follows which can boost anyone's game.

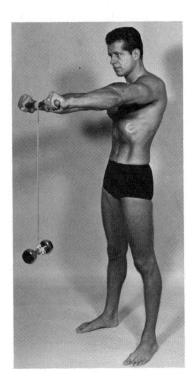

Using a stout string or twine, attach a weight to a piece of wood (a broomstick and steam iron would do nicely) and hold with arms straight in front of you at shoulder level, hands about a foot and a half apart. Roll stick forward until the weight winds to the top. Slowly roll down again. A beginner should start with five and increase gradually to 20.

Demaret says his legs were kept in condition by six days of golf a week for the 20 years he spent on the tournament circuit. Today he keeps them in shape by doing half-knee bends, using the edge of a straight chair as a stopping point. (See Page 33.) The average golfer can begin these in a series of 10 and increase until he is doing 25 at least three times a week.

3. Gary Player

This slight gentleman from South Africa has done more to popularize the muscular way to sub-par play than any other pro. Even his famous garb reflects his physical approach to the game. Black shirt and slacks, he claim, make him feel more powerful. This is psychological theory, but it is scientific fact that dark colors retain heat.

Player's problems in competing with the two other long-knocking members of golf's Big Three, Arnold Palmer and Jack Nicklaus, have led him to exercise more than any other golfer. Player decided long ago that he needed to beef up his shoulders, arms and wrists. By process of elimination he settled mainly on one exercise—the finger-tip pushup.

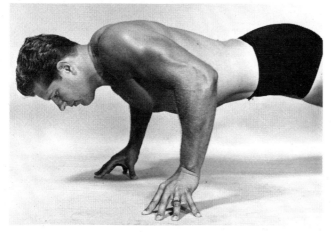

This is the same, in all save one respect, as the ordinary pushup. Brace your feet against a wall or heavy piece of furniture, keep legs straight and hips higher than shoulders at all times. Support your body on outspread fingertips, hands about shoulder-width apart. Lower your body until your chin is within two or three inches of floor an push up until arms are straight again.

This adaptation gets all the benefits of the standard pushup, with the important plus for the muscle in the forearms, wrists and hands.

Begin with five, if you can, increasing gradually to a goal of 20. Player at one time was doing three sets of 50 fingertip pushups daily, but he slacked off from fear they were making him muscle-bound.

After you win the Masters, you can worry about that, too.

Sex Exercise—Restoring That Old Zambola

Bring on that boy,
He'll be a toy
To Lola.
Just one more case
She can erase,
With that old zambola.

—A Little Brains, A Little Talent
(from Damn Yankees)

This chapter is, if you'll pardon the expression, the climax of the book. Its place of importance is due to my belief that sexual impotence in the American male has grown to epidemic proportions.

Furthermore, it is a crippling malady. The man who is impotent, even part of the time, suffers a blow to his ego that destroys his confidence in himself as a male. It is a failure that precludes happiness, and it can easily lap over into his professional life and reduce his ability as a wage earner.

Someone who prides himself on a detached intellectual view of life might term these reactions "extreme" or say they signify immaturity. Not so. The basic male function as procreator is the bedrock of manliness. Facing the loss of this function, a man is entitled to feel despair.

You can understand then why I term it a tragedy that so many men must suffer intermittent or permanent impotence *needlessly*. Fading virility is the motive, whether admitted nor not, of the majority of men who begin a program of exercises to regain physical fitness. The fellow who is frank enough to admit his reason has the battle half won before he starts. But in either event, in nine cases out of ten, his troubles will be cured.

A man's reluctance to disclose a record of impotence, even to his doctor, is understandable when you consider the social significance: it's supposed to be funny. Chaplin demonstrated how close pain is to humor, laughter is to shock. I wince when I hear a locker-room joke on the subject, something about a fellow who took 24 pills every hour instead of one pill every 24 hours, because I know that somewhere within any group of men there is one poor guy who is laughing to hide his humiliation.

There is a befuddling mountain of literature, both scientific and charlatan, on the subject of age-and-sex and failure in lovemaking. The causes are divided into two catagories: Organic and Psychological, both terrifying.

The organic reason, or alibi, is the more comforting to a man's self-respect, but it is proportionately rare. The mechanics of erection originate in the nerve system in the lower back, where the hip bones join the spinal column. Injury or disease may wreak damage that persists after you have recovered in all other ways. Leukemia, tuberculosis and anemia share impotence as a symptom. It is also one of the early signs of diabetes. A malfunctioning liver may loose an excess of female hormones to the body, causing "only" a decrease in sexual interest and power.

The Psychological causes bring us to the world of the head shrinkers. The suggestion that impotence originates in the subterranean recesses of your mind unleashes a chamber of horrors: You are a latent homosexual. You have an incestuous love for your mother. You hate your wife. You hate all women. And so on.

This is the underside of the rock a man turns over when he fails in bed.

Well, baloney!

When a guy is troubled by impotence, the cause is so elemental it would be laughable, if it weren't tragic: *He is simply too pooped to make love.*

The root of 90 per cent of sex failure is poor physical condition. The male's role of aggressor in the love act makes demands on the body which some men cannot meet. Either he is just generally weak 'and tired, or he lacks strength in the key muscular areas. A self-contempt for his physique can be another crippling factor—a psychic handicap because it relates directly to his manliness.

These are the physical shortcomings which open up the Pandora's Box of organic and psycho reasons for impotence. One incident of impotency leads to chronic impotency, long after the original problem has vanished. Failure breeds failure, because the *fear* of failure is its main guarantee. Which leads us back to the first problem, a man's confidence in himself as a man.

You may say, now wait a minute. I know old George over there who never had a muscle in his life and he is a heller with women. Maybe so. I am not saying that superb physical conditioning, bulging muscles and four-minute-mile stamina are *necessary* for a successful love life. (Even a satyr, however, could improve his record by improving his fitness.)

I am talking about the man who has a problem of impotence, or other sex failure, including premature orgasm or no orgasm at all. Most of this man's trouble is that he is just not strong enough. Furthermore, if he has a physical or mental flaw, *an increase in physical ability will overcome that flaw.*

My knowledge on this subject is entirely practical. Or, in the scientific sense, empirical. That's the scientist's word for finding an answer to a problem without the complex data leading to its solution. I have known increased physical prowess to work wonders in the sex lives of hundreds of men. For all the ones I know about, I believe there have been hundreds of others who have been rewarded in the same way.

What, then, are the Sex Exercises?

Almost any exercise, in its indirect way, is worthy of the term. An improved physique automatically boosts a man's confidence in himself as a male. I have seen such an improvement alter the flaws in a man's personality, add assertiveness, dignity, sociability, mature judgment, or other qualities he may have lacked.

But there are specific Sex Exercises which can restore that old zambola. Reflect on it a moment and you will see the logic: The sex act, as any other physical act, calls upon one area of the body, the midsection; and specific sets of muscles, in the lower abdomen and in the lower and middle regions of the back. The following exercises are directed at those targets.

Ideally, these routines should be part of a general conditioning program, as outlined in the first part of this book. At the least, they should be preceded by a few minutes of jogging and one or two exercises aimed at the shoulders, chest and legs.

But whether or not any additional conditioning is done, these Sex Exercises are vital.

1. The Bicycle Ride

This and the two succeeding exercises are designed to increase blood circulation in the pelvic zone. Wherever there is increased muscular activity there is increased blood flow, and this in turn nourishes the mechanism of erection, activated by nerves from the sacral portion of the spinal cord.

Lie on your back, lift your hips and support with your hands so that your legs, when straightened, are pointing directly at the ceiling. This is a matter of balance more than strength and is not as difficult a trick as it may first appear.

Now pump your legs as if riding a bicycle. The important movement is the thrust of each knee as you bring it downward to your chest. This thrust should be as deep as you can make it, because this is the main objective of the exercise, to massage and activate the lower abdomen and groin.

Taking care to thrust deeply with each knee, do the exercise as rapidly as you can, stopping on the count of 30. Increase gradually after the first few days in both speed and number, until you are doing a rapid 60, or 30 thrusts with each knee. For the first five weeks, ride this bicycle twice a day, then drop to one session per day.

2. Leg-Knee Squeeze

Lie on your back, raise right leg as nearly straight up as you can and grasp the right thigh in both hands, near the knee. Now, keeping the leg reasonably straight, pull the thigh toward you as far as you can. Hold for a count of three. Duplicate the exercise with the left leg. Begin with three repetitions, each leg, and increse gradually to 10.

Next draw your right leg toward you with bent knee, until your knee is as close to your chest as you can get it. Clasp the knee in both hands and press your thigh against your body. Hold for a count of three. Duplicate with left leg. Begin with three repetitions, each leg, and incrase gradually to 10.

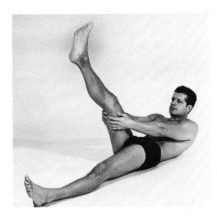

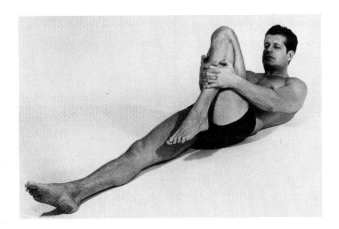

3. Double Knee Hug

Lie on your back and bring both knees toward your chest simultaneously. Clasp hands across your knees and pull hard against the abdomen. Hold for a count of five. Begin with five repetitions and increase gradually to 15.

4. The Pelvic Tilt

You must incorporate inner muscle action with the mechanical movements of this exercise. Assume the stance of a baseball outfielder, hands on knees. Put a sway in your back and take a deep breath, drawing in your abdomen. Now make a thrust forward from the hips, humping your back, and keeping your hands in contact with your knees. The sudden movement will tend to raise your upper body, but at least keep your fingertips in touch with your kneecaps.

It is on this thrust forward, this pelvic tilt, that you must call on muscle control. Tighten your buttocks and the sphincter muscle which shuts off the flow of urine. This double-flexing of two neglected muscles, which occurs at the same time of natural tightening of the abdominal muscles, is a very neat trick which takes practice to perfect.

Start with five and increase gradually to 20. Do not hurry this exercise. It takes concentration to achieve a good pelvic tilt.

5. The Rocking Chair Press

This is one violent step forward from the Rocking Chair Roll on Page 138. In fact, you should review the exercises for the back in that chapter before advancing to this one.

Lie on your stomach on a soft, flat surface and clasp your hands together in the small of your back. Lift the legs together as far off the floor as you can. Next lift your head and torso upwards as far as you can. Now alternately lift legs and torso in rhythmical fashion.

Begin with five lifts, both legs and torso, and increase gradually to 15.

6. The Two-Way Situp

This exercise should be approached with caution and with graduating strength. First work up to a level of 20 repetitions of the standard situp (see Page 19).

Now you are prepared to do the Twisting Sit Up and the Abdominal Press Sit Up.

Lie on your back and clasp hands behind neck. Raise torso upright and lean forward to touch right elbow to left knee. Recline again, raise upright and touch left elbow to right knee. Your feet, of course, must be anchored under a piece of furniture or held in place by a partner. Begin with six repetitions, three to each side, and increase daily by three to a goal of 12 to each side.

Next draw your feet toward your buttocks until your feet are comfortably flat and braced against the floor. Clasp hands behind head, raise torso and lean forward as close to your thighs as you can, holding for a count of two. Return slowly to reclining position and repeat. Begin with three repetitions and gradually increase to a goal of 15.

* * * *

I am putting it conservatively when I say these exercises will make a new man of you.

And that, after all, is the end idea in a program of physical fitness.

Your Aching Back! And How To Rebuild It

"Nagging" backache — a very apt and descriptive adjective. Men who are overweight and out of shape feel a sense of discomfort. But the poor guy with the inadequately conditioned back, he is in pain. At the least it is nagging, and for quite a bit of the day it nags like the point of a knife, spreading upwards from about three inches above the pelvis.

The reason for this malady is most often structural. It is the fellow with the long waist, the man who was slender in his youth and has become increasingly swayback as the years paraded past. He is most susceptible to back strain, which can be caused by almost any little thing — lifting a small bucket that is heavier than you think or, as we shall be reminded, planting a small tree.

Men of compact, or stocky, build may also suffer from backache, but it is rare unless a severe strain or accident has occurred.

The late John F. Kennedy, whose back ailments focused wide attention on this very democratic ache, had a longwaisted and limber physique. His troubles originated in a football injury when he was a freshman at Harvard. His back was more severely damaged when his PT boat blew up under him in the South Pacific. Years later, after he was elected to the U.S. Senate, this injury led to a dangerous spinal operation. Kennedy re-sprained his back planting a ceremonial tree in Ottawa in 1961. A wrong twist with a shovelful of dirt did the damage. This time the pain was so acute that he spent weeks getting around on crutches.

Aside from the commiseration offered by back sufferers every-where, the major result of these Presidential trials was widespread publicity about the treatment that reconditioned Kennedy's back. We can now benefit from the same methods to help any other afflicted sacroiliacs in the audience. Kennedy, of course, healed himself through exercise, and we shall see what kind they are.

The treatments were outlined by Dr. Hans Kraus of New York University at the request of Kennedy's personal physician, Dr. Janet Travell.

Kraus had been a particular student of back ailments and, with Dr. Sonya Weber of Columbia University Medical School, once conducted an experiment with a group of psychoanalysts, whose sedentary profession made them particularly vulnerable. In fact, all of·the men questioned had some degree of back ache, but the ones who were physically active had less pain than the others. Drs. Kraus and Weber prescribed exercises for 52 of the psy-choanalysts, and the results were so obvious that the experiment produced a basic premise: "Lack of physical activity is the major cause for low back pain. Exercise has both remedial and preven-tive value."

Let's examine the progressive stages of back exercises, beginning with the remedial, advancing to the preventive and ending with the toughening muscle builders.

1. Leg and Torso Stretch

Lie on your stomach with hands at sides, palms up. It's not necessary to lie on a hard surface. The idea is not to punish your stomach and chest, but to condition your back. Use your bed, if you wish. First raise the right leg as high as you can without discomfort. Try not to bend your leg at the knee. Hold it briefly at the peak of the raise, then lower. Next lift your left leg the same way. Now

138

move your head up and back as far as you can and lift your torso upwards. You will not be able to hold your torso at the peak of the raise for more than an instant. Next repeat the series, beginning again with the right leg. Start with three repetitions the first week, then increase to five for another week, gradually working up to 10.

2. The Curving Sit Up

Lie on your back with your heels drawn up close to your hips, feet flat. Anchor your toes under a heavy piece of furniture or have someone hold them. Fold your arms across your chest. In separate order, lift your head, neck, upper back and lower back up and forward until your forearms are as far forward of your knees as you can reach.

The separate lifting of head, neck, etc., brings more individual muscles into play. The final stretch forward with your forearms works the lowest muscles in your back. To return, reverse the process, attempting to place the lower back, upper back, shoulders, etc., on the floor in definite movements. This slow rhythm of the exercise is important to its effectiveness.

Start with three repetitions, twice a day. After a week, increase to five, and in succeeding weeks graduate to a goal of 15 per session. When you finally note new strength in your back muscles, you may move on to the next exercise.

(To relieve current back pains, do an easier variation of the curving sit up. Place two bedpillows, one in front of the other, sidelong on the floor against a wall. Place a third pillow sidelong on top of them and lean your back against this support, with heels drawn up and arms folded. Lean forward until your arms are as far in front of your knees as is comfortable, then return slowly to pillows, tightening your stomach muscles so that your lower back is first to press against them. Start with three repetitions, twice daily, and increase gradually to 10.)

3. The Rocking Chair Roll

This is an extension of the leg-and-torso stretch, and when you get it going good your body will be moving like a rocking chair arm.

Pick a soft surface or you are likely to develop corns on your belly button.

Lie on your stomach, arms at sides, backs of hands pressed to floor. First, raise both legs together as far as you can without flexing knees. Next, lift your head up and back and raise your torso as far as you can. Keep raising legs, head and torso in rhythmical succession.

Begin with three, twice daily, and after a week increase to five repetitions. Then gradually reach a goal of 15 per session. Do not let the exercise overtax you at any time. Stop every now and then for a 20-30-second rest and let yourself go completely limp. Always take such a rest after completing the exercise.

4. The Reverse Sit Up

This one is for post graduates, or men with strong but fat backs. The complaint about persistent rolls of fat across the small of the back at the beltline is rare, but in some physiques this excess is too stubborn to be removed by anything less than an exercise directed at that specific area.

You will need a helper to get the main benefit from the reverse sit up. He must anchor your feet firmly to the floor by gripping your ankles.

Clasp your hands across the small of your back, lift your head and torso as far off the floor as you can and held for a count of two. The degree of height you achieve will increase over a period of weeks as you continue the exercise. Start with three repetitions, and increase one a day, if you can, to a goal of 20. After a week at 20, you may cut the sessions to three times a week.

Watch out for your return trips when you lower your torso and head to the floor again. Unless you are doing the exercise on a bed the face-landing could lose a few teeth for you.

* * * *

Two further words of caution: The back reacts violently to changes in temperature on the muscles. Be wary of heating pads, especially while sleeping because you may turn away from the pad during the night and expose your sweating back to cold air. After an exercise session avoid the flow of air-conditioning units. Take a warm shower or bath and towel yourself dry vigorously.

If you now have back pains, consult a doctor and get his approval for the exercises I have suggested here. Backaches have hundreds of causes, each difficult to pinpoint. Extreme cases call for a brace, or even surgery.

When a man has recently sprained the muscles in his back, he even has difficulty getting out of bed in the morning, much less thinking about exercising. Even diathermy treatments may not help. But the muscles need to be flexed if he is to rid himself of the pain. The solution is miraculous in its effectiveness: He should get himself immediately to a swimming pool. The free buoyancy of the water supporting his body removes the normal demands being made on the muscles. Even the most painfully sprained back will be suddenly soothed. The patient should tread water in the deep end of the pool and alternately arch his back, as if in a swan dive, and hump it by drawing knees to chest and hugging his legs tightly. This painless flexing of the muscles will restore them in one-fourth the time it would take the pain to simply wear itself out. The session in the pool need not be more than 10 or 15 minutes, repeated several days in a row. Each time the sufferer will leave refreshed and relaxed.

If your back is healthy, start exercising now to keep it that way. "Oh, my aching back!" is no joke, and it doesn't have to be more than a figure of speech.

Isometrics: Six Seconds To Added Strength

The popularity of the isometric exercise is the only new development in body conditioning within the last three thousand years. It's easy to understand why it has captured the imagination of people everywhere.

It takes only *six seconds to* perform any isometric exercise. And the results are astounding.

The principles of isometrics, of course, have been used haphazardly before now. Physical therapists prescribed them, out of necessity, for patients immobilized in bed or a wheel chair. But it wasn't until a German scientist, after the war, began experimenting and recording statistics on the effect of these exercises that they became practical for everyone, healthy or ill.

The word itself, from the Greek, means equal (iso) measure (metron). The basic principle is that if you cause a muscle in your body to tense to its utmost, the muscle will automatically be strengthened.

There is no motion involved. You simply cause the particular muscle to work against an immovable object. The force you exert is reversed, in equal measure, to your muscular system.

Within a matter of a few weeks you will have converted flab into firm flesh, weakness and lassitude into strength and energy. The routine is so successful it is being used by National Football League athletes, golfers, bowlers, skiers, and even weightlifters. The latter especially find it helpful when they get to a "sticking point" in their training and find themselves unable to advance beyond a certain weight in repetitions. They knock off and go to the isometric bar, and in a few days they are strong enough to soar to a new level on the weights.

But let's understand, first, what isometrics do not do. They do not affect your body weight appreciably. They do not increase your stamina. They are no help to the healthful conditioning of your cardiovascular system.

But they are excellent and wondrous supplements to your regular program of calisthenics and weight loss campaign. For one thing, they will certainly reduce the size of your waist line — by strengthening the muscles that hold the stomach in its rightful place. And by adding strength everywhere on your body, they restore a vigor and zest for life that you most certainly have been missing.

Here are the basic isometric exercises, none of which require any equipment not available in your home:

Doorway Press

1. For lower back muscles, biceps, and backs of thighs: Stand in doorway and press palms of hands upward against doorjamb. Your

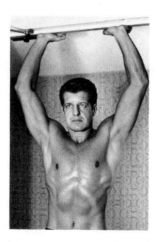

Doorway Press

arms should be slightly flexed, legs straight. Stand on a low footstool, if necessary, to get the desired position. Now thrust upward with both arms for six seconds of peak effort. You will feel the muscles in your lower back tensing. Next flex your knees so that your arms are straight. Thrust upward as before, for six seconds, this time using your thigh muscles to generate the pressure. One repetition per day of each exercise is all that's necessary.

2. For upper back and shoulders: Stand in doorway and place palms against doorjamb on each side of you. Push outward with both arms for six seconds. This is an excellent prescription for slumping posture.

3. For latissimus dorsi muscles at your side near back of armpit: Stand in doorway facing one side of the doorjamb. Spread your legs about shoulder-width apart for balance and leverage. Place palm of right hand flat against wall beyond edge of doorjamb and press for six seconds toward the left. Repeat using the left hand. Forearm should be horizontal to the floor. This exercise will build the V-shape torso by increasing the muscles in your back from the shoulders to the waist.

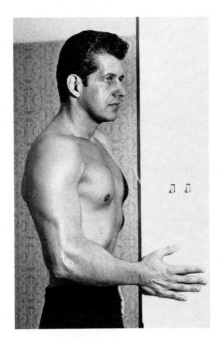

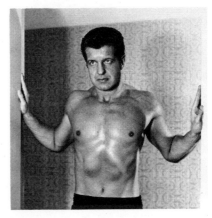

Doorway Press

4. For front of thighs and for calves of legs: Stand in doorway with your back against one side of the doorjamb and your right foot pressed about waist level against the opposite doorjamb. Exert full pressure for six seconds. Repeat with left leg.

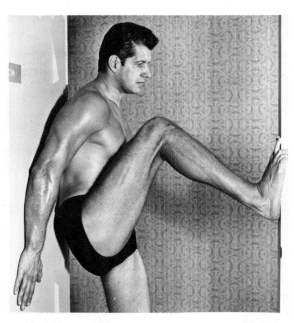

Doorway Press

The Wall Press

1. For tricep muscles along back of upper arms: Flex knees slightly and place your back flat against a wall, arms extended downward and palms flat to wall. For six seconds press against wall with the palms. You will feel the muscles along the backs of your arms tensing. This will firm a major area for flab.

2. For arms, back and shoulder muscles: Stand erect facing wall, feet about shoulder-width apart, arms extended downward and slightly outward from your body. Stand close enough to the wall so that you will have to turn your face to one side. For six seconds, exert pressure against wall with the palms of your hands.

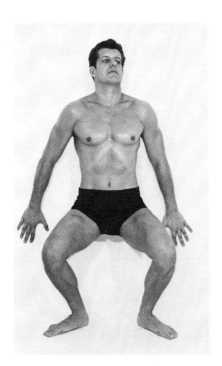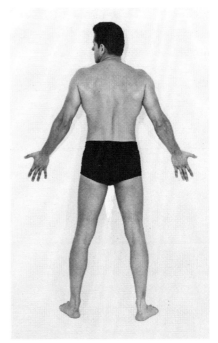

The Wall Press

The Towel Lift

1. For forearms, wrists and biceps: Grasp an ordinary bath towel at both ends behind your back. Stand with feet shoulder-width apart and flex knees to that your thighs are nearly horizontal to the floor. Pull upward on the towel with both hands so that the towel is taut underneath your thighs. Exert maximum pressure for six seconds.

2. For arms and shoulders: Grasp bath towel with hands about 12-18 inches apart. Resisting with right hand, pull upward with left hand for six seconds. Switch hands and repeat. (This is an exercise that you can repeat again and again whenever you are lolling on the beach or around a swimming pool.)

3. For legs and wrists: Sit on floor, grasp ends of bath towel and place your feet together to push outward against the loop of the towel. Your feet should be eight to 12 inches off the floor. The balance is

tricky at first, but not difficult after a few tries. As always, exert maximum pressure with your legs, resisting with a pull on the towel, for six seconds.

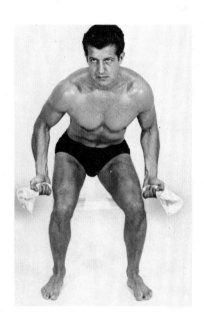
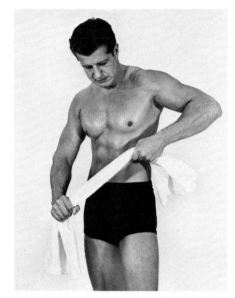

Towel Lift

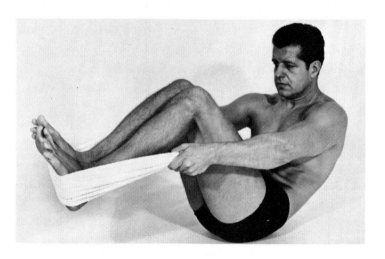

Waist Reducers

1. For upper and lower abdomen: Stand with feet shoulder width apart and rest hands on knees. Exhale completely after taking deep breath. Now try to touch your backbone with your stomach, tensing as hard as you can for six seconds.

2. For lower abdomen: Lie on your back with palms pressed flat against floor. With legs straight, have your ankles underneath the edge of a heavy coffee table or bed. Try to lift legs up through the bed or table, exerting pressure for six seconds.

3. For upper abdomen: You will need either an isometric bar which can be lowered to the desired level, or an assistant to hold you immobile. Lie on your back with arms extended above head and begin to raise torso to upright position. The bar, or helper, should stop you after torso is about 12 inches off floor. Exert pressure at this position for six seconds.

*   *   *

These are only the rudimentary isometric exercises to get you started on the correct idea. It should be obvious to you by this time that you can work any muscle in your body if you isolate it properly against an immovable object. This routine can be a boon to your efficiency at pastime sports, and some kind of isometric exercise can be performed throughout the day — at your desk in the office or at the steering wheel of your car.

Good Grooming

*Next to clothes being fine, they should be well made, and worn easily:
For a man is only the less genteel for a fine coat if in wearing it, he
shows a regard for it, and is not as easy in it as if it were a plain one.*

Lord Chesterfield

While the cosmetics industry is believed to have many of the answers
to good grooming for the male in this decade, cosmetics alone—no
matter how much we come to use or even depend upon them—will
never make the compleat well-groomed man.

What is good grooming and where does it apply?

There are five areas that you have to take into consideration if you
wish to appear well groomed: the hair and scalp (and we have already
discussed this in previous chapter); the skin in general, including the
nails; the face in relationship to shaving; the body itself; and clothing
—as Lord Chesterfield has pointed out in the quotation at the opening
of this chapter.

Let's discuss these specifics in a little detail:

Scalp and hair we have already discussed in some detail. If, after
all, you are still having troubles (most likely because it is already too
late to rectify the situation) you can take comfort in the fact that cos-
meticians feel scalp problems and probably baldness will soon become
a thing of the past. By the end of this decade, they predict, everyone's
hair will be longer and healthier-looking due to advances in preparations now being developed.

What about hair pieces? There is no doubt that a hair piece added to a thin or bald situation improves the appearance. There are a number of ways in which such hair patching can be done and this should be thoroughly investigated by you if you decide to go this route.

The skin is very important to good grooming. Those portions of your skin that are readily visible—the face mostly—tend to indicate just how clean you are and how much you think of yourself. And, in this context, don't forget your nails.

It isn't necessary to have your nails manicured every time you go to the barber shop. You can keep them neatly filed—use an emery board rather than a nail file or nail clipper, because this keeps the nails from cracking—and use of cuticle remover once a week or so will keep your hands looking presentable. As far as keeping the nails clean, there is no reason why you can't carry a nail file in your pocket and make sure that excessive dirt is kept from piling up under your nails and giving your hands a dirty, ugly look.

A good way to prevent dirt from piling up under your nails is to use a nail brush daily and make sure that soap gets under the nails with the brush. This prevents oiliness from developing in these particular crevasses and, therefore, prevents dirt from accumulating in the oily areas.

Soap and water is still the best cleaner of all for the skin. When it comes to the face, such a cleansing should be done two or three times daily at minimum. Hot water will open the pores and soap will clean them out. Then, after thorough hot water rinsing, a cold water rinse will close the pores—or you could possibly even use an astringent to tighten up the skin in this way—and keep dirt from accumulating in your skin.

Tanning, though not to excess, keeps the skin looking healthy. A little sunlamping on a daily basis should keep the tan even throughout the year.

As far as your body skin, we will discuss this a little further on.

The shave is a daily ritual which may be boring to some. Electric shavers are becoming more capable of doing a good job, and you may find that one type does a better job for you than another. Test them and find out.

For men who use safety razors, the new finishes on blades has made this daily job easier to do and take. There are also new preparations that make the job less onerous.

The old bugaboo about shaving against the grain seems to have lost some of its proponents. It may well be that when you start to shave against the grain (perhaps after having shaved with the grain), ingrown hair will develop. But, after treating them—as I outline below—you will find that the facial hair will accommodate to this style of shaving and this problem will not recur.

The body should be treated the same way as the face. A shower at least once daily with the hot/cold water treatment as for the face is highly recommended. A *loofa* sponge, obtainable at most druggist shops, does wonders for the skin, especially when you rub it over those areas of the back that are the least accessible.

Attention should be paid to such things as ingrown hairs, blackheads and excessive oiliness. The loofa and showerings should ease the blackhead problem. Ingrown hairs should be carefully plucked with tweezers and then the area should be bathed with Zephirin Chloride to cleanse the skin and prevent infection.

The body should smell clean. Some men have problems of excessive perspiration. This can be most uncomfortable. And the odor is a discomfort to those near you.

New products cope with both problems—find the one that works best for you. Watch out for some ingredients which may irritate you. If that happens, shift to another deodorant until you find one that does not irritate your skin.

Drinking more water during the day than you usually do will help dilute the strength of your perspiration and therefore make the odor less powerful. Try that trick if body odor continues to be a problem.

Your dress acts like a table of contents to a book. The way you appear tells what's inside more surely than anything else. Of course, there are untidy geniuses, but we are all not geniuses so let's not hide behind untidiness.

No matter what your financial state is (and therefore how expensive your clothes or how recent in fashion) there is no excuse for untidy dress. Shoes can always be shined, pants pressed, etc. Wash-and-wear clothing makes it easy today to keep underthings clean (and freshly worn daily). You would be surprised how underwear and socks worn more than one day can give off an odor that others can smell—and deodorants don't cover that kind of smell.

Wash-and-wear shirts, too, are easy to keep clean—and touch them up with an iron so that your shirt-front looks neat.

Ties on which you've dropped food can be kept clean of stains—as can other clothes—with a variety of cleaning methods that are inexpensive and easy to do. Even lighter fluid will clean off a grease spot from tie or jacket—so there is no excuse to look like a slob.

The man of the decade should be lean, tanned and healthy...young in both outlook and perspective.

Addendum

PROTEINS: The food element from which all body tissue is built, and therefore the most important ingredient in your diet. An abundance of protein is necessary for growth. The most efficient suppliers of protein: egg yolk, cheese, milk, yogurt, liver, kidney, brain, sweetbreads, roasts, chops, steaks, soya beans, nuts, wheat germ, and cottonseed flour. Less efficient, but still plentiful suppliers of protein: dry beans, lentils, dry peas, corn, rye, gelatin and egg white.

Inadequate protein in your diet will lead to pale color of blood, low blood pressure, fatigue, poor muscle tone, faulty posture, and low resistance to infection and disease.

CARBOHYDRATES: The sweet and starchy foods that are most easily converted into fat by your body function — bread, cereals, potatoes, spaghetti, etc. The danger — as far as weight-gain can be termed a danger — is in adding saturated fats to the carbohydrates. That is, butter with potatoes. This will more than double the calorie total: $1/3$ pound of baked potato is 125 calories, and $3/4$ ounces of butter totals 188 calories, for a grand total of 313.

VITAMINS: The classification of substances necessary to life. Herewith a brief description of each vitamin:

Vitamin A — Always found in association with fat in the animal body. It is stored in the body and does not require daily replenishing.

Milk, egg yolk, liver, cod-liver oil, lettuce, carrots, spinach, turnip tops are rich in Vitamin A. White bread lacks it.

This is the vitamin that provides a glowing complexion.

Vitamin B — Now known to be at least six different vitamins, including Vitamin B-2, which has become known as Vitamin G. The lack of Vitamin B-1, or thiamin, causes irritableness and nervous disorders, and in extremity, beriberi. It is found abundantly in corn or wheat germ, yeast and rice polishings, as well as such common foods as milk, fresh fruits, whole grain cereals, fresh vegetables and modern enriched flour and cereals. It must be replenished daily.

Vitamin G — This is the antipellagric vitamin, and unlike B-1 it is not destroyed by heat. It is abundant in milk, liver, yeast, lean beef, green, leafy vegetables and bananas. Lack of Vitamin G brings about stunted growth, loss of weight, soreness of eyes, mouth and nose.

Vitamin C — Chemically, absorbic acid, a vital ingredient to your all-around health, which will be satisfied by regular consumption of citrus fruit in all forms, juice and fresh, and by tomatoes, particularly the plum-size tomatoes. Absence of Vitamin C brings about scurvy. The body is unable to store Vitamin C for any length of time, so keep it coming.

Vitamin D — In childhood, this ingredient prevents rickets. The most natural source in sunshine striking your bare skin. Fish and other sea foods are the most abundant edible sources. Vitamin D has been added to milk, and particularly to skim milk.

The other vitamins, such as P, K, E, are almost automatically included in your everyday intake of food, unless you are in a prisoner of war camp.